OVERCOMING OVERACTIVE BLADDER

Your Complete Self-Care Guide

Diane K. Newman, RNC, MSN
Alan J. Wein, MD

New Harbinger Publications, Inc.

Publisher's Note

Care has been taken to confirm the accuracy of the information presented and to describe generally accepted practices. However, the authors, editors, and publisher are not responsible for errors or omissions or for any consequences from application of the information in this book and make no warranty, express or implied, with respect to the contents of the publication.

The authors, editors, and publisher have exerted every effort to ensure that any drug selection and dosage set forth in this text are in accordance with current recommendations and practice at the time of publication. However, in view of ongoing research, changes in government regulations, and the constant flow of information relating to drug therapy and drug reactions, the reader is urged to check the package insert for each drug for any change in indications and dosage and for added warnings and precautions. This is particularly important when the recommended agent is a new or infrequently employed drug.

Some drugs and medical devices presented in this publication may have Food and Drug Administration (FDA) clearance for limited use in restricted research settings. It is the responsibility of the health care provider to ascertain the FDA status of each drug or device planned for use in their clinical practice.

Distributed in Canada by Raincoast Books

Copyright © 2004 by Diane Newman and Alan Wein
New Harbinger Publications, Inc.
5674 Shattuck Avenue
Oakland, CA 94609

Cover design by Amy Shoup

ISBN 1-57224-339-2 Paperback

Printed in the United States of America

New Harbinger Publications' Web site address: www.newharbinger.com

06   05   04

10   9   8   7   6   5   4   3   2   1

First printing

Contents

Acknowledgments

Many people helped during the writing of this book, and we are thankful to them. We are enormously grateful to our editor, Spencer Smith and the entire New Harbinger publishing team. Our thanks to both Estelle Covely and Michael Newman who reviewed the chapters through this writing process. Last, but not least, to our patients, who have allowed us to care for them. We hope this book expands your understanding and encourages you to seek solutions.

To our families for all their understanding and patience.

—Diane & Alan

Introduction

Emily has been a teacher for the past fifteen years. A couple of years ago, she started noticing that she had to leave her fourth-grade class before the morning recess because of a strong need to urinate. Initially, she was able to delay the urge, but as time went on her urgency became more severe and was occurring more often. She started asking her teaching assistant to take over the class, but the assistant was only there on Mondays and Thursdays. Emily mentioned it to her gynecologist, who told her what she was experiencing was common. He didn't suggest what she should do, but then Emily didn't really ask. Emily is thinking about quitting her job and going on disability. She doesn't know what else to do.

Emily has a fairly common problem called *overactive bladder* (OAB). OAB is a bladder control problem that has four basic symptoms: *bladder urgency*, a strong desire to urinate that is usually accompanied by *urge urinary incontinence*, the unwanted leakage of urine on the way to the bathroom. A person with OAB can also have *frequency*, which is urinating more than eight times a day, and *nocturia*, awakening at night to urinate. OAB is a problem for over seventeen million Americans and is an extremely costly problem for consumers and the health-care industry. In terms of dollars and cents, OAB annually costs the U.S. health economy between sixteen to eighteen billion dollars. Millions of Americans suffer the embarrassment, inconvenience, and serious medical consequences of uncontrollable urges to urinate and the need to frequently use the bathroom. Although some people seek treatment, you may be one of the many that attempt to hide your condition from your family, friends, and even from your doctor and other medical providers. You may be like the majority of people who believe that nothing can be done to help their condition and that bladder problems like OAB are simply a part of aging that cannot be changed. Increased urgency, frequency, and urge urinary incontinence negatively affect your quality of life. Most importantly however, overactive bladder and its underlying cause can now be treated very successfully, improving your life and your overall health. However, effective treatment cannot reach you unless you acknowledge that you have an OAB problem and seek help.

Until recently, overactive bladder was a silent subject. It was rarely disclosed by people suffering from it or openly discussed within families, and many times it went undiagnosed or ignored by nurses and doctors. During the past decade the treatment and care of incontinence and especially overactive bladder has undergone a revolution. Media attention has brought overactive bladder into the public spotlight. Through newspaper, magazine, and TV coverage of the human and economic toll of overactive bladder, people with this condition are learning that they need not suffer alone. *Help is available.* Self-help groups such as the National Association for Continence (NAFC) and the Bladder Health Council of the American Foundation for Urologic Diseases (AFUD) have contributed to public awareness. Information is also available in cyberspace—on the World Wide Web at www.seekwellness.com and on Internet discussion groups.

We've written this book for you if you suffer with overactive bladder. We want you to have the basic information about your OAB condition so you approach your problem with understanding and the ability to make decisions about your treatment. This book will also be useful for those who have a family member or close friend dealing with OAB and caretakers for people suffering from it. Reading *Overcoming Overactive Bladder* will help you take the first step to conquer and cure the condition by providing:

- ♦ A complete picture of what overactive bladder is and how it occurs

- ♦ An explanation of the bladder and how it functions

- ♦ A list of related bladder conditions

- ♦ A review of how doctors assess the problem

- ♦ Information about dietary habits, bladder retraining, and exercises that are effective

- ♦ Details about current medications that can control and even stop your symptoms

- ♦ Descriptions of surgical procedures that can provide relief in persons who have failed all other treatments

♦ Lists of devices that can contain urine leakage or can provide you with personal security if all else fails

Usually, the first barrier to seeking help for people with OAB is the difficulty in admitting that the condition exists. Since overactive bladder usually starts out as a slight problem, slight urinary urgency and frequency, most people don't view it as a problem right away. When the condition gets worse, which it's apt to do, you may be ashamed and lack the courage to tell your doctor or even those closest to you about your experience. The longer you wait to address the problem, the worse it gets—sometimes bringing unnecessary health-care complications and costs. If you suffer from OAB, don't let shame and embarrassment stop you from getting help and taking care of yourself. Be proactive and seek help. Consider what Emily did.

When Emily confided in a friend about her anguish over her OAB problem, her friend suggested she make an appointment with a local urologist. The urologist suggested that Emily try a medication that would decrease her urgency and frequency by causing her bladder muscle to relax. He also told her to make an appointment with his nurse practitioner who would teach her some bladder-retraining tips to also help her urgency. Emily left his office feeling optimistic that she could control her bladder and continue teaching.

OAB can be devastating, but it can also be controlled, helping you get back to your normal and productive life. This book will provide the information you need to recognize your overactive bladder problem, empower you to seek help, and to find a solution. Take that first step and learn about OAB and what *you* can do about it.

Chapter 1

The Problem of Overactive Bladder

What is Overactive Bladder?

Because conditions affecting the urinary system and bladder have often been uncomfortable or "taboo" subjects in the past, overactive bladder (OAB) has been under-reported and under-diagnosed. OAB is a medical problem that has been shrouded with silence and ignorance and has thus been inadequately treated and poorly addressed by medicine, despite the substantial impact on individual health, self-esteem, and quality of life. If you suffer from OAB, it's important that you have all the facts, so let's take a closer look at what we mean by overactive bladder. Consider Laura's story.

> Laura is very distressed. She never had any bladder-control problems until she turned sixty-four, but now she can't control the urge to urinate. Sometimes the urge is so strong that she feels she won't make it to the toilet if she doesn't run. The other day Laura had a real "urinary accident." Driving home from the mall, she got a strong urge to urinate. She parked the car in the garage, grabbed her shopping bags, and rushed to the door. She fumbled with her keys, couldn't get them in the lock, and the urge became so strong that she completely "lost it." Laura wet through her pants. She was so glad that at least she'd made it home and wasn't stuck at the mall.

Laura has most of the common symptoms of overactive bladder; urinary urgency with urge urinary incontinence. The large muscle in the bladder known as the "detrusor" is integral to storing urine. If you have OAB, your detrusor muscle becomes too active, causing you to want to urinate more often. The muscle contracts more often than normal and at inappropriate times, leading to urine leakage. Due to this, people suffering from OAB typically have to empty their bladders frequently, and when they experience a sensation of urgency, may leak urine if they're unable to reach the toilet quickly or if the sensation of urgency is very strong. In some cases, the cause of OAB may be neurological (nerve) damage from certain medical conditions such as stroke or multiple sclerosis, but in most cases the cause isn't known.

More on the Symptoms

For more detailed definitions of these important OAB symptoms, we can turn to an international medical organization called the International Continence Society (ICS) that has provided the following definitions.

Urgency. This is the sudden, intense, and often overwhelming desire to urinate that is difficult to delay. People report that the urgency is so great that they need to rush to the bathroom frequently, but when they urinate, it's usually only in small amounts. In most cases, the person doesn't have enough time to reach a toilet and involuntary urine leakage occurs.

Urge urinary incontinence (UUI). When you don't have time to make it to the bathroom, UUI is often the result. It is the involuntary leakage of urine accompanied by or immediately preceded by urgency. Urge urinary incontinence is also commonly referred to as "loss of bladder control." This is due to involuntary or "overactive" bladder contractions that cause the pressure in the bladder to exceed the pressure in the urethra sufficient enough to cause urine loss. The amount of urine lost may be large (greater than three ounces), or the bladder may empty completely. Even though your bladder is full, you may not get any early urges telling you to urinate. People with UUI will complain that the need just hits all at once, and the urine just "gushes" out. Laura has a common sequence of urgency often referred to as "key in the lock" or "garage-door syndrome"—strong urges to void as soon as one returns home and attempts to open the front door or garage door, regardless of how recently the bladder was emptied. A person is very aware of the need to urinate and yet can't seem to get to the toilet before having an accident. When the incontinence occurs at night it's called "nocturnal enuresis" or "bedwetting." In many cases, these symptoms are related to overactivity of the bladder, but they can also be caused by other forms of bladder dysfunction. Also, certain activities or events may trigger sudden urgency and urine leakage. Some common ones include:

♦ Hearing running water

♦ Washing dishes or clothes

♦ Placing your hands in warm water

♦ Anxiety or stressful situations

♦ Exposure to cold (for instance, leaving a warm house to go out into the cold)

♦ Seeing a bathroom sign

Frequency. If you're urinating more than eight times during the day, you're experiencing frequency. You may feel you urinate too often. Of the three symptoms, frequency is the most common symptom reported in persons with overactive bladder, and urge incontinence is the least.

Nocturia. This is when frequency occurs at night while you're asleep. Usually your sleep is disturbed because you have to awaken two or more times at night because of the need or urge to void.

The Magnitude of Overactive Bladder and Incontinence

OAB can vary from person to person, from day to day, and can occur rarely or frequently. If you experience urine loss, the amount can be a few drops or as much as a cup. At some time in our stressful, active, and hectic lives, most people experience an incident of severe urgency with subsequent incontinence. But when that incident develops into a pattern of urgency with increased urinary frequency with or without urine leakage and the pattern is serious enough to disrupt your lifestyle and daily routines, it becomes an overactive bladder condition. Having an overactive bladder may cause you to:

♦ Start "toilet mapping," which is when you habitually look for toilet locations and plan your daily activities based on knowing where toilets can be easily reached;

◆ Experience disturbed sleep and daytime irritability due to waking up to go to the bathroom two or more times during the night;

◆ Repeatedly leave important meetings because of frequent trips to the bathroom;

◆ Pass up invitations to socialize with friends and family because of the embarrassment of having to visit the bathroom regularly or the fear of having an incontinence accident;

◆ Only sit in the aisle seat in public transportation, on planes, in places of worship, or at movies so you'll be able to leave quickly to find a bathroom;

◆ Always carry a spare set of clothing in case of an incontinence episode;

◆ Wear dark and baggy clothing to disguise disposable pads or the signs of urine leakage;

◆ Carry a bottle or some type of container in the car in case you need to void while traveling long distances;

◆ Withdraw from sexual intimacy to avoid the anxiety and embarrassment caused by urine leakage during lovemaking;

◆ Avoid or stop exercising, like jogging, because of the fear of being too far away from a bathroom;

◆ Silently endure a condition that no one is talking about and falsely believe that there is no hope or treatment.

OAB is a set of symptoms that define a bladder problem, and its causes are unknown. OAB is seen more often in women, than men, and though it's not a disease, it can be a chronic or long-term problem. Although most often seen in adults, it can disable even the young. It is feared by those who suffer from it, goes unrecognized by many medical providers, and generally is misunderstood by the public. Medical providers estimate that OAB with incontinence ranks among the ten most common chronic medical conditions and affects more Americans than any other single medical problem, condition, or disease (Wein and Rouner 1999). Research published in the Journal of the American Geriatrics Society has shown that OAB is a major cause of falls in the elderly, thus leading to increased chance of medical complications like hip fracture (Brown 2000).

Rose has leaked urine, from time to time when she coughs or laughs, since her last baby was born forty-five years ago. It wasn't really an inconvenience, because it was only a few drops each time and she could use a small pad to contain it. If her husband noticed that she had a problem, he never mentioned it. About ten years ago, when she broke her hip and had surgery to replace it, she began to lose urine on her way to the bathroom. It soaked through her pad to her skirt, and Rose has been worried that her daughters will discover her secret. Sue, her good friend and neighbor, had the same kind of bladder problem and her sons sent her to a nursing home in a nearby town because they felt unable to help her. Rose doesn't want that to happen to her.

Like Rose, you may be experiencing OAB due to a variety of factors including aging, loss of the estrogen hormone after menopause, adverse effect of medications, and physical and mental disabilities that cause nerve damage. As you age, your bladder loses its firm shape, shrinks, or drops from its correct position in the pelvic area. It tends to relax, increasing urgency and frequency and sometimes allowing urine to dribble or flow out in a stream. Usually a person is unaware that urine leakage is about to happen. Although you may not be able to control all the factors that lead to your condition, you *can* gain control of overactive baldder.

Who is Experiencing OAB?

Mary, a nurse, had a very disturbing conversation with her friend Helen. Helen was helping her seventy-six year old mother wash a load of clothes and noticed that the clothes had a strong urine odor. Helen was worried that her mother had a bladder problem. Mary asked Helen if she had discussed her concerns with her mother, and Helen explained that her mother is a very private person who has always been concerned about her personal health. Helen felt that if her mother wanted to discuss a bladder control problem, she would bring it up herself and would be very upset if someone in her family asked her about it.

Does Helen's story sound familiar? Maybe you have an older family member or friend with these same problems. OAB is more often seen in the older adult, with one out of three women and one out of five men over the age of sixty-five experiencing incontinence. Many more have the bothersome OAB symptoms of urgency and frequency. A survey conducted in the United States called the NOBLE (National Overactive Bladder Evaluation) study found that 63 percent of adult men and women had OAB *without* incontinence and 37 percent had OAB *with* incontinence. In a survey of six European countries (Milsom 2001), frequency was the most commonly reported symptom (85 percent), followed by urgency (54 percent) and urge incontinence (36 percent).

Although a wide range of therapies and management techniques are available to help you if you're experiencing OAB (at least 80 percent of treated persons improve), you may be like most people who don't seek treatment for their overactive bladder. A telephone survey of a sample of American adults demonstrated that fewer than 40 percent of patients with symptoms of OAB reported ever seeking treatment for the condition, and only 44 percent had mentioned their symptoms to a medical provider in the previous twelve months. The fact that people do not seek treatment for OAB is not unique to Americans—it happens throughout the world. A similar survey in Europe found that 40 percent of patients with symptoms of OAB had not mentioned the problem to a medical provider, and in Asia, only 21 percent of women with OAB sought treatment.

Even in cases where OAB is severe enough to cause urinary incontinence, only half of the afflicted persons mention their symptoms to a medical provider. People who decided to discuss their incontinence with a doctor waited an average of three years, with some waiting as long as five years (Ricci et al. 2001). Many persons accept OAB as only a minor problem, or they find the topic too embarrassing to discuss with medical providers. A survey conducted in England demonstrated that 81 percent of people who had not mentioned their incontinence condition to their doctor did not want treatment or help, and two thirds were too embarrassed to even mention their condition.

The most common reason for not seeking treatment for OAB is the mistaken belief that successful treatment is unavailable. This misconception is shared by many medical providers. A recent survey showed that a majority of primary care doctors saw "lack of available and effective treatments" as a major barrier to their patients. A discussion about overactive bladder and incontinence with many doctors in this survey felt that current treatments have less than a 50 percent chance of resulting in significant improvement. Another survey done at the same time indicated that over 86 percent of patients who did discuss their overactive bladder and incontinence with their doctor were unhappy with the outcome, and in many cases, were told by their doctor that incontinence was simply a normal part of aging. This is not surprising, as a review of medical-claims data of insured persons who reported OAB indicated that people were not receiving successful treatments, such as drug therapy. These discouraging responses are very unfortunate, since behavioral and drug therapy now exist that can completely eliminate or significantly reduce urgency, frequency and urge urinary incontinence in over half of the persons treated, with substantial improvement occurring in an even greater percentage.

Separating Fact from Fiction

There are many untruths, myths, or fiction about OAB and urinary incontinence. It's important to separate the facts about this condition from the misconceptions so you can make informed decisions. Below we've listed the common myths about OAB and provided the truth about each. See if any of these beliefs have taken up residence in your head.

"I'm Just Getting Old"

Bodies do change with age, but overactive bladder is *not* an ordinary or inevitable part of this aging process. However, there are physical and medical factors that affect a person's bladder sensations and awareness:

♦ The loss of the hormone estrogen in women during menopause may cause a thinning of the tissues surrounding and supporting the bladder and pelvic area. This results in a loss of support for the muscles of the bladder and pelvis leading to urgency and frequency.

♦ Enlargement of the prostate gland in men may inhibit the complete emptying of the bladder, resulting in urgency and urinary "dribbling."

♦ Decreased bladder capacity in older adults may cause urinary urgency, leading to frequent voiding and incontinence.

♦ Susceptibility to urinary-tract infections increases with age and predisposes some seniors to symptoms of urgency, frequency, and incontinence.

♦ Arthritis and diabetes, common ailments contracted as a person grows older, may result in urinary incontinence.

Diabetes can affect the nerves to the bladder muscle, preventing it from emptying completely. Arthritis can affect your ability to make it to the bathroom in time.

◆ Chronic medical conditions requiring multiple medications may further predispose seniors to urinary symptoms.

◆ Vision and mobility changes as a person ages and may impair an individual's ability to get to a toilet in time.

◆ Many seniors may have difficulty using toilet facilities. When a person has urgency and encounters a public restroom with a four-digit combination lock, opening the door may be an insurmountable obstacle.

"Nothing Can Be Done about It"

This is one of the saddest misconceptions about OAB because it can be treated successfully, with cure and improvement rates of 85 percent. Most people are unaware that help is available. Among the current ways to manage OAB are:

◆ Diet and lifestyle modification

◆ Bladder retraining

◆ Kegel or pelvic-muscle exercises

◆ Medications

◆ Surgery

◆ New technology in devices to help with management

With careful treatment and attention, OAB caused by diseases such as diabetes may be completely reversible. Hand in hand with the fiction that nothing can help, is the denial by some that they, indeed, have a bladder-control problem. Many see their condition as only short-term, a situation that will probably resolve itself. For many people, it's very difficult to deal with the reality of OAB or any bladder-control problem. If shame, fear, and outside pressures force you into a defensive posture, you end up hurting yourself and your health.

"I'll Need Surgery"

Seniors are very worried that if they discuss their OAB with a doctor, surgery will immediately be suggested as the cure. If you have OAB, surgery should only be performed if all other treatments have failed.

What OAB Costs

For the past several years, Janet has found herself going to the toilet frequently to avoid "not making it in time." She puts paper towels and tissue in her underwear for protection. Last week she had an accident that saturated her underwear and skirt. Janet feels she may need to buy some of those incontinence pads she's seen in the drugstore, but she is a widow on a fixed income and doesn't think she can afford this added expense.

Because OAB is a common condition in women and men of all ages and particularly prevalent in the elderly, it has serious implications from a health-economics perspective. With rising health-care costs and a growing population of older adults, we all need to be concerned about the cost of OAB. The world's population is expected to expand to 7.5 billion by 2020 (from 5.7 billion in 1995). By 2020, there will be 44 percent more people over the age of sixty-five and, for many, OAB will be a debilitating condition. It's expected that OAB-related costs will increase with the aging population. There will also be increased awareness of OAB, coupled with the availability of better treatments and changes in treatment-seeking behavior. More people will be seeking help for their OAB symptoms in the primary-care setting, by primary-care doctors, internists, and nurse practitioners. These factors, together with a better understanding of intangible costs, are likely to produce a magnitude of change in the costs associated with OAB.

Other costs contributing to the economic burden associated with OAB and incontinence includes treatment of the conditions related to OAB, including skin breakdown and infection resulting from rashes and pressure sores, urinary-tract infection, anxiety, depression, low self-esteem, and social isolation. The financial burden is further compounded when considering the fact that older patients with poor mobility, coordination, and vision appear to be at increased risk for falls and other accidents because of their bladder condition. These cumulative expenses reveal the extensive nature of the economic burden on the health-care system—and possibly on you if you or a loved-one is dealing with OAB. Though the financial impact of OAB can seem daunting, it can provide even more incentive to make use of the treatment options available—from your doctor and from this book—to help improve your symptoms.

We have provided an overview of OAB, defining the common symptoms, its magnitude, and its high costs, but to truly understand your symptoms, you need to learn about your bladder and how it works. Move on to chapter 2 to learn more.

Chapter 2

Understanding
The Bladder

In order for you to understand overactive bladder, you need to understand the urinary tract system, how it works, and what happens when it doesn't work.

The Urinary Tract

Everyone has a urinary tract system, upper and lower. Figures 1 and 2 (on the following page) show the organs involved. The upper portion normally consists of two kidneys, each with a long, thin, muscular tube attached (called the ureter) that carries the urine from the kidneys to the bladder. However, you can live a perfectly normal life with just one of each. The lower urinary-tract system contains the bladder, urethra, sphincters, and, in men, the prostate gland.

Function of the Kidneys

The *kidneys* are one of the body's primary filtering systems, eliminating waste from the blood and creating urine. The kidneys and the ureters are in the upper urinary-tract system. The kidneys are bean shaped organs located on either side of the spinal cord behind the lower ribs. The kidneys filter wastes from the blood, resulting in what we call urine. This filtering allows the body's basic functions—temperature, blood pressure, blood sugar, etc.—to remain in balance. *Nephrons*, a set of very complex tube-like structures in the kidneys, delicately balance filtration, reabsorption, and secretion of the body's fluids. The kidneys filter roughly forty-two gallons of blood a day, but only about one percent of the blood's salts and water are passed out of the body in urine. Urine consists of

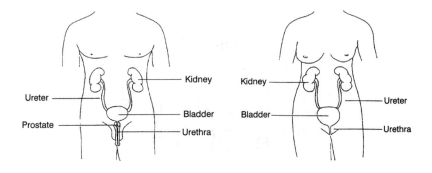

Figure 1: Front View of the
Male Urinary System

Figure 2: Front View of the
Female Urinary System

approximately 95 percent water and 5 percent dissolved wastes
(urea, creatinine, and uric acid).

The kidneys constantly send urine to the bladder through the
two ureters, which are approximately nine inches long. The urine is
forced through the ureter by contractions of the muscles in the
ureters and with the aid of gravity. Urine enters your bladder, where
it's stored until a certain volume is reached, causing your bladder to
contract, forcing the urine into the urethra and out of your body.

Understanding the Bladder and Urethra

To maintain bladder control or continence, normal functioning
of the lower urinary tract, bladder, urethra, sphincters, and pelvic
floor muscle support is imperative.

*Joe's bladder controls his life. Ever since he was diagnosed
with BPH (enlarged prostate), he has had to learn the location
of every restroom at the mall when he shops with his wife.
Joe finds himself avoiding unfamiliar places. Before driving
from his house to see his daughter, he always uses the
bathroom, even if he doesn't need to. Not surprisingly, Joe,
like most people, doesn't really understand how his bladder
works.*

The *bladder* is a hollow muscle that functions like an elastic
storage tank, moving urine through a drainage tube called the urethra. Located in the pelvis behind the pelvic bone, the bladder
changes shape according to the amount of urine it contains. When

empty, it resembles a deflated balloon. As the amount of urine in your bladder increases, the bladder becomes somewhat pear shaped and rises into the lower abdomen. The bladder is fully movable except at its base, or neck, where it becomes part of the urethra. Urine is temporarily stored in the bladder, until it's passed through the urethra and out of your body.

The bladder wall consists of three layers: mucosa, submucosa, and muscle. The *mucosa* is the innermost layer and the submucosa lies immediately next to it. The *submucosa* supports the mucosa, supplies its blood vessels with nutrients and lymph nodes that help remove waste products. The muscle, also called the *detrusor,* is a thick layer of smooth muscle that expands to store urine and contracts to expel it. At the base of the detrusor muscle is the bladder neck or *trigone,* a triangular area located within the bladder wall. According to some scientists, the trigone may contain most of the sensory nerves of the bladder (see Figure 3). The bladder is often referred to as just the detrusor muscle.

Overactive bladder is characterized by uncontrolled or involuntary contractions of the detrusor muscle. These uncontrolled bladder contractions occur at low bladder volumes and give rise to frequent sensations of urgency (a strong feeling of the need to urinate). If these muscle contractions cannot be suppressed or inhibited, or the person does not reach a toilet in time, then urine leakage may occur—the symptom known as urge urinary incontinence. Of course, when you suffer from increased urgency, your bladder isn't being used to capacity, resulting in an increased frequency of urination.

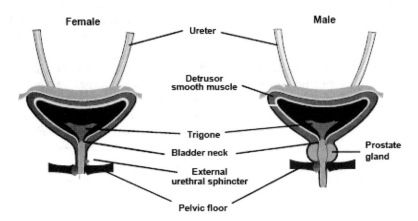

Figure 3: Front view of the Female and Male Bladder

The *urethra* is a small, slender tube, leading from the neck of the bladder to the outside of the body. In women, the urethra is short—only one-and-a-half inches long—and is embedded in the front wall of the vagina. The opening of the urethra is called the *urinary meatus* and is located between the clitoris and the vaginal opening. Because the clitoris, vaginal opening, and urethra are located so close to each other in a very small area, the urethra is not easy to find. A woman may need to use a mirror to help locate her urethra.

In women, the vagina is continuous with the bladder base and with the urethra. The mid to lower vagina is supported by connections to the pelvic floor muscle.

A man's urethra is about eight inches long. It leaves the bladder and passes through the prostate gland, the pelvic muscle, and the length of the penis, ending at the tip or glans of the penis. The prostate is a walnut-sized gland located at the base of the bladder, surrounding the urethra like a doughnut. The portion closer to the urethra can enlarge, causing obstruction. The main function of the prostate is to manufacture secretions that become components of semen.

The Importance of the Urinary Sphincters

Regulation of the storage and emptying of urine from the bladder is controlled by the internal and external urethral sphincters. A *sphincter* is a ring-like band of muscle fiber that closes off natural body openings such the anus and the urethra. Sphincters are supposed to stay tight or closed without a person needing to think about it. When sitting, standing, or walking, urine does not leak out of the bladder or urethra because the sphincters keep the urethra closed. The sphincter relaxes when messages are sent from the nerves and the brain to the pelvic floor muscles.

The external sphincter lies below the internal sphincter. It is a muscle that can be consciously controlled. The external sphincter's voluntary contraction allows for urethral closing during instances when there is more pressure in your abdomen, like when you sneeze, cough, or laugh. These sphincter muscles work closely together to control the various stages of bladder filling and emptying. (See Figure 4.) The muscles around the bladder neck automatically expand and contract, holding urine in or letting urine out of the bladder. As the bladder fills, the nerves tell the muscles to keep the sphincter contracted and no urine is released. You are unaware of this message; it happens with no conscious action on your part. However, at a certain point the internal pressure of the bladder

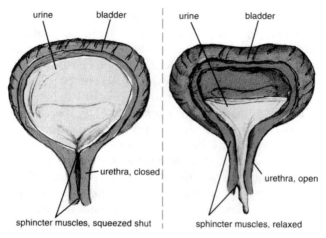

Figure 4: Parts of the Bladder Control System

increases to a level that leads to stretching of the bladder wall, and a message is sent to the base of your brain through your nervous system. Your brain then sends a message to the detrusor muscle in the bladder to automatically relax your internal sphincter. The external sphincter now consciously tightens, and you feel a strong urge to urinate. When urinating, normally you relax your external sphincter muscle.

The Support by the Pelvic Floor Muscles

The bladder neck and the urethra are supported by a series of interconnected muscles called the *pelvic floor muscles*. The pelvic floor contains a meshwork of muscles that run from the tailbone at the base of your spine to the pubic bone in the front of your pelvis. This muscle group are referred to as the *pubococcygeus* (*pubo*: pubic bone, which is the anterior attachment of the muscle and *coccygeus*; coccyx, which is the posterior attachment) or *levator ani*. You can refer to this as the *pubococcygeus* or *levator ani* muscle. A man's prostate gland, as it grows, provides some support for the pelvic floor. As a woman reaches maturity, the hormone estrogen helps keep her bladder, urethra, and muscles in the pelvic floor healthy and assists in maintaining good pelvic floor muscle tone. As a woman ages and goes through menopause, her estrogen level drops, causing a loss of muscle support in the pelvic area.

The pelvic floor is not a rigid platform, but a strong, flexible muscular structure, often described as a "hammock" of muscle. The pelvic muscle consists of striated muscle fibers that are under voluntary control and can be exercised. We'll be learning how to strengthen these muscles later in the book. The pelvis supports the spinal column, which is attached to the rear of the pelvis. The bladder, urethra, rectum, and, in women, the uterus, lie above and within the pelvic area. The pelvic floor surrounds, suspends, and anchors the pelvic organs, helping them remain in place. These muscles contract and expand during voiding and bowel movements and distend during and contract after childbirth. The pelvic floor muscles can be used during sexual intercourse for the stimulation of a partner's penis. When infection or physical trauma damages the pelvic floor, the firmness and health of pelvic muscles and nerves are affected, causing organs—the bladder neck, urethra, or the uterus—to drop or sag. This puts unnatural pressure on pelvic floor muscles, causing conditions such as incontinence or infection.

The Role of Your Brain and Nerves

In simple terms, continence and incontinence is really controlled by your brain.

The bladder, urethra, and pelvic muscles receive messages from the brain by two systems of nerves, called sympathetic and parasympathetic. The *parasympathetic* releases a chemical called acetylcholine that stimulates receptors (called cholinergic receptors), in the body of the bladder, causing the detrusor muscle to contract and allow the bladder to empty. The *sympathetic nervous system* has what are called alpha adrenergic and beta adrenergic chemicals. The alpha adrenergic substance affects receptors in the trigone of the bladder and receptors in the internal sphincter. The beta adrenergic substances stimulate receptors in the bladder body that results in smooth muscle relaxation of the bladder wall.

In the pelvic area, the pudendal nerve provides vital support for the pelvic muscles. The pudendal nerve has two branches—the anterior branch goes to the urinary tract and the posterior branches to the intestinal tract, or the rectum. The nerve is like the trunk of a tree sprouting branches of nerves out to the urinary tract and the rectum. The pudendal nerve controls the external urinary sphincter. These neurons are located in the sacral nerves (found in the lower spinal cord) called Onuf's nucleus, which has a high concentration of serotonin and norepinephrine neurotransmitter receptors.

As an infant, a person has little control over the urge to void. As the brain, muscles, and nerves mature, a "Bladder Control Center" develops. Located in the base of the brain, the Bladder Control Center coordinates sphincter relaxation during voiding. Urinary continence results when each system receives and correctly responds to the messages to void or not to. Overactive bladder results when there is a breakdown in communication between the Bladder Control Center, the bladder, and the sphincter. This breakdown may be caused by a mental or a physical impairment or by a disease like stroke, Parkinson's Disease, or Multiple Sclerosis.

The Path to Normal Urinating

The lower urinary tract is essentially a high-volume, low-pressure system. As long as the pressure within the urethra remains higher than the pressure within the cavity of the bladder, you will be continent or dry. Even when the bladder is full, it's elastic enough to accommodate additional fluid without causing pressure within the bladder to exceed or overcome urethral pressure. The bladder holds between twelve and sixteen ounces of urine. Normally you will feel the urge to urinate when the bladder contains about eight to ten ounces of urine, about as much fluid as in a can of soda. There really are no "normal" urinating patterns. Patterns that do exist range from every four to six hours to every six to eight hours. Seniors over sixty-five may urinate every three to four hours and at least once during the night.

The urge to urinate is an uncomfortable feeling that makes you want to empty your bladder. Usually it indicates your bladder is full. However, if you have frequent voiding and incontinence, the bladder may not be full, but may be contracting and producing the urge.

The lower urinary tract system contains the bladder and the urethra. This system can be compared to a plumbing unit, with the bladder functioning as a "tank" and the urethra as a "hose." The urethra is always closed or "kinked" so that urine does not escape and your external sphincter keeps the urethra closed. The urethral (or external) sphincter muscles surrounded by the pelvic floor muscles remain contracted to prevent urine release. When the bladder fills to capacity, nerves send messages to your brain causing the internal sphincter to open and the first sensation to urinate occurs. As urinating is voluntary, you make a conscious decision to go to the toilet or to delay urinating. When you decide to urinate, the internal sphincter relaxes, pressure in the bladder increases and assists in pushing the urine into the urethra, the external sphincter relaxes and urine is passed out of the body.

Bladder Changes with Aging

Carolyn has just turned seventy-two and is starting to feel old. She finds herself going to the bathroom once an hour and getting up twice at night to urinate. Sometimes the urge comes up so quickly that she's afraid she won't get there if she doesn't run for it. Many times she puts a washcloth between her legs just in case she has an accident. When Carolyn told her family doctor about the problem, he just shook his head and cautioned her to be careful not to fall when she is rushing to the bathroom.

Instead of being aware that their bladder is filling and may soon need emptying as younger people are, seniors are often unaware until their bladder is almost full and they need to urinate *now*. To an active, mobile person, no matter what age, locating toilet facilities may be an inconvenience. To an immobile adult, a senior citizen, or an individual with an unstable bladder, "warning time"—the time between the realization of the need to urinate and the actual release of urine—is critical. Delaying urination can often result in involuntary urinary "accidents."

Another age-related change is that bladder capacity is diminished. The detrusor muscle tends to shrinks in size or capacity and cannot hold as much urine as it did in younger years. Therefore, seniors get the urge to void with lower bladder volumes and urgency may be more intense and occur suddenly.

Two-thirds of seniors' daily fluid intake is excreted at night. This is because the kidneys make urine faster and more efficiently when you're lying down and at rest. The heart pumps more blood to the kidneys faster in a prone or supine position and the kidneys are able to filter wastes more efficiently. Seniors may need to use the bathroom one or more times a night, these trips often produce falls and broken bones, especially in hips, legs, or arms. Seniors who do not completely empty their bladders make many trips to the bathroom during a night.

Now that you understand how your urinary tract works, let's discuss other related bladder problems so you can better understand what you're experiencing.

Chapter 3

Related Types of Bladder Disorders

If you have OAB, it's important to distinguish your problem from other urinary or bladder conditions. Although urge urinary incontinence, a symptom of OAB, is the most common type of incontinence in older persons, stress incontinence is very common in women under the age of sixty-five, and many persons will have symptoms of both types, which is called "mixed incontinence." Identifying the type of incontinence you're suffering from and other common bladder disorders that may be affecting you will help your medical provider select the most appropriate treatment. In this chapter, we discuss the different types of urinary incontinence and other related bladder conditions seen in both men and women.

Other Types of Urinary Incontinence

In addition to urge urinary incontinence, there are several other types of incontinence. They are:

- ♦ Stress

- ♦ Overflow

- ♦ Functional

- ♦ Reflex or neurogenic (nerve related)

In young adults each can occur alone, but older adults and seniors often suffer from a combination of stress and urge incontinence (mixed incontinence). Some types of incontinence may be transient (for instance, occuring because of an infection) and are the result of changes in the bladder or urethra or due to damaged pelvic muscles and nerves. Chronic or long-standing incontinence occurs because of persistent abnormalities of the structure or function of the lower urinary tract, including:

♦ Bladder overactivity, or the bladder contracting when it should not

♦ Bladder underactivity, or the bladder failing to contract when or as well as it should, causing the bladder to stay full and some "overflow" of urine to occur

♦ Urethral obstruction, usually due to an enlarged prostate or stricture (narrowing of the urethra)

♦ Urethral incompetence, where the resistance of the sphincter mechanism is too low, resulting in urine leakage with effort

Stress Incontinence

Michelle, a fifty-four-year-old career woman, just finished experiencing menopause. She was advised by her doctor to begin an exercise program to keep in shape and strengthen her bones. She enjoys a daily run, but has started to leak drops of urine while running. Her friend Allison said, "Don't worry, it's normal for a woman your age. That's what those thin panty-liner pads are for."

Michelle is experiencing *stress urinary incontinence* (SUI), which is leakage of a small amount of urine with physical exertion or activity. SUI is all about urethral support and resistance and increased pressure or stress on the bladder. As the stress or pressure increases, the bladder neck can't handle it because the pelvic support network isn't strong enough. The muscles in the pelvic floor area and the surrounding tissues are the key to urine control. Laughing, coughing, sneezing, running, jumping, exercising, lifting, sitting, standing, and other strenuous physical activities cause a rise in abdominal pressure, leading to SUI. These activities increase pressure on your abdomen, causing pressure on your bladder. Another complaint you may have is losing urine when getting up from a chair. This happens because your abdominal muscles are pushing down on your bladder, causing SUI.

Stress urinary incontinence usually produces only small amounts or "drops" of urine leakage. However, the amount of leakage may change, depending on the specific activities that cause the urine loss and how severe your sphincter problem happens to be (Newman 2003). Severe SUI can even occur during minimal activity, such as changing positions in bed, or the leakage may be unrelated to an activity. Causes of SUI include these:

♦ Weakened muscles and tissues in the bladder outlet and the pelvic floor cause the bladder and urethra to sag or shift. Abnormal urethral movement, called *hypermobility,* can occur during physical activity or exertion. The urethra can't control the flow of urine, and small bursts of urine leak out of the urethra.

♦ As women age, many develop intrinsic urethral sphincter dysfunction (ISD), which is urine leakage due to a damaged or weakened sphincter. Typically, more women than men experience this kind of stress incontinence—six out of seven people with this problem are women. Because of pelvic anatomy, the pelvic muscles in men are rarely stressed and stretched, while childbearing stretches and relaxes a woman's pelvic floor and may damage nerves in the pelvic area and tissue in the bladder's neck. Norton and colleagues (2002) have reported on a soon-to-be-released antidepressant called duloxetine that prevents the release of serotonin and norepinephrine, which are chemicals or neurotransmitters found in the external urinary sphincter. Duloxetine may help close a weak sphincter and prevent SUI.

♦ Prolapse of your pelvic organs can be a cause of SUI. The position of the uterus, bladder, and bladder neck within the pelvis has a direct effect on the control of urine. You may have heard your mother or a friend speak of a "fallen uterus" or "fallen bladder." Usually women with this problem will start a pattern of urinary frequency because they believe a stress accident is more apt to happen with a full bladder.

♦ SUI in men can be caused by prostate surgery, especially for cancer and lost function in their urethral sphincter muscle.

Overflow Incontinence

Allen, who is sixty-eight years old, noticed that his urine stream had become slower and less forceful and never seemed to stop. Just when he thought he was done, some urine would dribble out, sometimes dripping on the floor. Allen's wife was always complaining about the urine on the floor around the toilet. His doctor sent him to an urologist, who found that Allen's prostate was blocking the tube that carries the urine from his bladder. His urine dribbled because the tube had narrowed.

Overflow incontinence is caused by blockage in or an obstruction around the urethra, causing the bladder to empty incompletely. If you have overflow incontinence, you dribble small amounts of urine throughout the day but feel like your bladder never really empties. When you go to the bathroom, you have difficulty starting your urine stream and once started, the stream is weak. Because the bladder never gets to empty, the muscle gradually stretches and stretches until it can't empty completely. In overflow incontinence, the person cannot empty their bladder completely but rather urinate in small amounts—the overflow urine. As the bladder is not emptying, the bladder muscle enlarges because it is working harder to try to empty. Think of the bladder muscle like a balloon. If you don't let the air out and keep filling it up, it will get larger. If overflow incontinence goes untreated, the urine that stays in the bladder can become infected, often spreading to the entire lower and upper urinary tract. In severe cases of overflow incontinence, the urine can back up into the kidneys, creating a dangerous medical problem. The causes of this type of incontinence include the following:

♦ An enlarged prostate in men that surrounds and blocks the urethra can prevent the bladder from emptying. The bladder becomes so full that it "overflows," and urine dribbles out.

♦ Prolapsed (sagging or dropped) pelvic organs in women can compress or "kink" the urethra, preventing urination.

♦ A stricture or scar tissue in the urethra can also block urination.

♦ Certain neurologic disease such as diabetes can affect nerves to the bladder muscle, preventing emptying during urination.

♦ Drugs such as pain killers, antidepressants, and smooth muscle relaxants may increase the capacity of the bladder, but they dull the sensation of the need to urinate and may reduce the ability of the muscle to contract normally.

♦ Trauma or injury to the nerves in the spinal column can affect the nerve supply to the lower urinary tract. Damaged bladder nerves and tissues can reduce the bladder's ability to contract and release stored urine. All of these problems can cause urinary retention (incomplete bladder emptying) and overflow incontinence.

Functional Incontinence

Frances is eighty-two years old and lives in a two-story home in Philadelphia. Her first floor has a living room, dining room, and kitchen. Bedrooms and the bathroom are on the second floor. In the morning, a nurse's aide comes to Frances's house to help get her bathed, dressed, and downstairs. Frances spends most of her day sitting in her living room until her niece comes home at 7 P.M. to help her get ready for bed. When Frances has to use the bathroom, she has a hard time getting up her carpeted steps and is very fearful of falling. Many times she is incontinent before she reaches the bathroom on the second floor.

This type of incontinence can occur if you're unable to get to a bathroom or are unwilling to use toilet facilities because of decreased mental awareness, loss of mobility, or personal unwillingness to go the toilet. It's felt that over 25 percent of incontinence found in hospitals and nursing homes is functional in origin. Common factors contributing to functional incontinence include the following:

♦ Decreased mobility or dexterity can cause difficulty in getting to the bathroom and removing clothes.

♦ Environmental barriers such as inconvenient bathroom or toilet equipment, stairs, the lack of handrails, and narrow doorways that don't accommodate wheelchairs or walkers can also hinder you in getting to the bathroom.

♦ Mental and psychosocial disability can cause a lack of awareness of the need to urinate and confusion over the location of the bathroom or individual toileting habits.

Reflex Incontinence

If you have a birth defect such as spina bifida or a spinal cord injury, you can develop reflex incontinence because you may not have the normal sensation to urinate and/or your bladder contracts involuntarily (a "neurogenic" bladder). You will either have your bladder contract without the sensation to urinate, causing incontinence or incomplete bladder emptying. Bladder emptying will occur at unpredictable times and in response to volume or other stimuli. Damage to nerves in the spinal column, complications of surgery, and other spinal problems prevent the transfer of nerve impulses from your bladder to your brain and back to your bladder. When these messages are disrupted, you have no indication of a full bladder. Certain urinating techniques can improve bladder emptying if you have some component of neurogenic bladder with retention. They include the following:

♦ If you don't have any spinal cord injury, you can find a "trigger" to initiate a bladder contraction. One common method is called "suprapubic tapping," which involves drumming the abdomen overlying the bladder. The application of rhythmic tapping is thought to produce multiple nerve impulses to stretched nerve receptors in the bladder wall by way of discharges (impulses) from the nerve reflex arc. The best suprapubic triggering technique is to tap the area over your bladder (called the suprapubic area) rapidly seven or eight times, stop three seconds, and repeat. Other trigger mechanisms include pulling your pubic hairs, stroking your abdomen or inner thigh, and digital anal stimulation. Your medical provider may want you to experiment to discover which technique works best and most easily.

♦ Double voiding may be effective and involves voiding twice during each trip to the bathroom. You simply urinate, stand up, wait one or two minutes, sit back down on the toilet, and try to urinate again.

Lower Urinary-Tract Symptoms

Older men may develop a variety of bladder disorders often referred to as LUTS (lower urinary-tract symptoms). These are usually related to an enlargement of the prostate gland. Men with prostate enlargement can develop "bladder outlet obstruction," which can lead to incomplete bladder emptying as the enlarged prostate causes narrowing and compression of the urethra. The prostate gland normally becomes larger with age and hormonal changes, and by the age of sixty most men have an enlarged prostate.

Aside from simply getting older, prostates can grow bigger or become irritated in different ways and for various reasons.

Prostatitis is the inflammation (swelling) of the prostate gland caused by either a bacterial infection or by the backup of prostate secretions within the prostate gland. Men will experience symptoms of frequency, urgency, and discomfort when urinating.

Benign prostatic hyperplasia (BPH) is a non-cancerous enlargement of the prostate gland. The prostate may enlarge to a size where it causes significant compression of the urethra. A result of this is that the bladder muscle has to work harder to carry out its mission of emptying urine. Over time, as the bladder muscle enlarges, the overstretched bladder is not able to contract at all or may contract weakly and with great difficulty. The bladder muscle may lose its flexibility and be unable to adequately store urine. The obstruction may also be associated with the development of bladder overactivity, or BPH may cause no symptoms. If obstruction occurs, the first symptoms may include:

♦ Urinary frequency

♦ Urgency

♦ Nocturia

♦ Hesitancy—a delay when starting to void

♦ A weak or interrupted voiding stream

♦ A continual feeling that the bladder is not empty

Prostate cancer can also cause narrowing and compression of the urethra but less commonly than BPH. The most accurate way to diagnose prostate cancer is through a blood test (PSA) and digital rectal examination during which the physician can feel whether a nodule (a firm or hard area) exists. The American Cancer Society recommends a digital rectal exam and PSA every year in men over fifty. Symptoms of prostate cancer include:

♦ A weak or interrupted stream of urine

♦ OAB symptoms of urgency and frequency

♦ The inability to urinate

♦ Hesitancy

♦ Hematuria (blood in the urine)

♦ Pain or burning on urination

♦ Continuing pain in the lower back, pelvis, or upper thighs

Unfortunately, symptoms of prostate cancer often occur late in the disease. After prostate cancer surgery, men may experience SUI for the first six months. Those men who have radiation or seed therapy for prostate cancer may experience urgency and frequency.

Prostate cancer surgery is called *radical prostatectomy* and is when the prostate gland and the cancer is removed through a surgical procedure. Radiation therapy is when radiation is delivered through a machine that emits a beam of radiation from outside of the body through normal body tissue to reach the cancer. Radiation is usually given five days a week for seven to eight weeks. Seed therapy is when tiny pellets of radioactive medication are placed in the middle of the cancer (in this case, the prostate gland), where they give off very small amount of low-level radiation continuously for around one year.

Infections, Cystitis and OAB

"I can't make it. It comes out too quick," complained sixty-six-year-old Joan. Joan was referred to the continence nurse practitioner because she had lost her bladder control after a recent hospital stay for a heart attack. Joan told the nurse practitioner that she has a history of bladder infections and cystitis. Joan had a catheter in her bladder while in the hospital, and it was removed before she was discharged. Since she's been home Joan feels that her urine "just gushes out." When the nurse tested Joan's urine she found that Joan had a bladder infection. Joan was given antibiotics and her urgency and incontinence problems stopped once the infection cleared.

An infection in the urinary tract (UTI), often called cystitis, is most often due to bacteria in the urine. The bacteria irritate the lining of the bladder mucosa and submucosa, causing frequency even if there is only a small amount of urine in the bladder. A UTI is seen more often in women than in men because a women's urethra is shorter and germs have an easier time and a shorter distance getting from the anus to the urethra. Approximately 50 percent of women will develop a UTI during their lifetime. UTI is more common in older women because of changes in the urinary tract that come with age and less efficient immune systems.

Infection can also cause urgency, urinary incontinence, and occasional pain or burning when voiding. Infection can cause an increase in bladder contractions and overactivity. Recurring infections may lead to a decrease in sphincter tone resulting in urine leakage. In younger and middle-aged adults, medical providers usually spot UTI immediately because the person will complain of burning sensations, frequent urination, fever, and lower-back pain. Urinary incontinence is often a senior's only symptom of an infection.

To determine the presence of a UTI, a urinalysis is done, testing for bacteria in your urine. If there is bacteria, your urine will be sent for a culture. If an infection is found, it's treated with antibiotics and in many cases, incontinence and other bladder symptoms will be resolved. If a person has frequent UTIs, vitamin C (ascorbic acid) may prevent recurrent infections. Women also report that cranberry juice or cranberry tablets may help, and the benefit may exist because cranberry juice or tablets reduce the bacterial adherence to the bladder wall. Causes of UTI include:

♦ Kidney or upper urinary tract infection

♦ Poor personal hygiene. Women should carefully clean themselves after each bowel movement, wiping front to back, so that bacteria from the rectum won't travel to the vagina and opening of the urethra.

♦ Vaginal douching and cleansers that can upset the normal balance in the vagina and can lead to an infection

♦ Wearing tight pants that can trap moisture and create a favorable environment for infections

♦ Using perfumed soaps, bubble bath, and talc powder, rough, perfumed, or colored toilet paper

♦ Using feminine hygiene or menstrual pads for urinary protection rather than wearing incontinence pads, which are designed to absorb urine. It's important to change your pads when they become wet with urine.

♦ The spreading of bacteria during sexual activity. An infection may be passed between partners, and sexual activities may bruise the urethra or cause swelling and inflammation in the vaginal area.

Interstitial cystitis (IC) is a bladder disorder that can be a severe, debilitating, and chronic disorder. IC is found mostly in women between thirty and fifty years of age. Caucasians comprise 94 percent of IC patients, with middle-aged Jewish women being the most commonly affected. However, many men previously diagnosed with certain forms of prostatitis actually have IC.

If you have IC, you have a bladder wall that is tender and easily irritated, leading to uncomfortable symptoms. When most medical providers think about cystitis, infection of the bladder comes to mind. That is because the most common form of cystitis is caused by bacteria and is aptly called *bacterial cystitis*. IC, on the other hand, does not appear to be related to infection. Women with IC complain of severe urinary frequency (up to fifty times per day), urgency, nocturia, dyspareunia (painful sexual intercourse), lower abdominal and pelvic pain and pressure, and depression. In men, slow urinary stream and pain at the tip of the penis, the groin, or in the testicles may be symptoms. Symptoms can worsen with certain foods or beverages.

IC generally begins gradually and becomes progressively worse. The symptoms may go away for a while (remission), but usually come back again. Symptom flares may be connected to the menstrual cycle. Spontaneous remissions may occur, but unfortunately, symptoms often return weeks to months later. Urinary incontinence is rarely associated with IC. The exact cause of IC is not really understood, but may include a variety of causes such as chronic infection of the bladder, lymphatic disease, autoimmune disorders (the body's defense system turning on itself), and even psychological disorders.

IC can have a devastating effect on the person's ability to function in every aspect of life. Often the pain is unbearable, and you may be unable to leave your home, causing you to isolate yourself from others. Frequency and nocturia can lead to chronic sleep deprivation and depression.

Now that you understand the different types of incontinence and related bladder problems, let's discuss the effect of OAB on your everyday life and how OAB impacts you, your family, and your friends.

Chapter 4

The Ramifications of Overactive Bladder

Overactive bladder is both a community health problem and a personal crisis. The consequences of both OAB and UI are shared by doctors and nurses and by your family and friends. There is also a broader impact, extending to environmental effects and rising health-care costs. This chapter will explore the effect of OAB on your life and detail who is at risk for developing OAB.

How It Affects You Personally

Assessment of quality of life are critical for conditions such as OAB, which often go untreated and have little or no impact on overall morbidity and mortality. The symptom of incontinence in people with urgency and frequency has significant physical, psychological, and social implications that include restriction of recreational activities, depression, loss of self-esteem, and sexual dysfunction. If you have OAB, you probably score lower in all quality-of-life categories than friends who are your same age and gender. Moreover, you'll probably be more emotional and less socially active.

If you are experiencing incontinence with urgency and frequency, your symptoms will have a greater impact on your life. Results from the National Overactive Bladder Evaluation (NOBLE) study, a U.S. screening program of 7,000 adults with symptoms of OAB, showed that there is a reduced quality of life and increased use of coping behaviors in those suffering with OAB (Stewart 2001). Quality of life is worse in those persons with OAB and incontinence than in those with OAB without incontinence. You may find that your urinary leakage is more distressing than do those people with other types of incontinence, especially those with stress incontinence. There are several reasons:

- ◆ Urge incontinence is less predictable.

- ◆ It typically results in a much larger volume of urine loss.

- ◆ Unlike stress incontinence, urge incontinence often causes problems at night, resulting in a loss of sleep and sometimes the need to change wet nightwear and bedding.

You should never underestimate the psychological impact of OAB, particularly if incontinence exists. Incontinence is more than just a hygiene issue, as you may find it difficult to socialize or communicate normally, placing a greater burden of care and emotional support on those who are closest to you. You may suffer the consequences of your symptoms for years, believing that treatment for OAB is not effective or that the symptoms are an inevitable part of the aging process. Do not just accept your OAB—seek help. There are successful treatment options available.

OAB, Incontinence, and Social Dysfunction

Kathryn has leaked urine from time to time, when she coughs or laughs, for many years. It had always been in small amounts and not a major concern. Recently, she went with her friends on a bus trip to the casinos in Atlantic City. It was a two-hour drive and Kathryn started having urgency that got progressively worse. The urge became so uncontrollable that she started to lose urine as she got off the bus. She was able to hide this from her friends, but she won't be going on any more of those trips.

If you have an overactive bladder, you may find that you're isolating yourself from your friends and family and will go to great lengths to hide your problem. You may reduce the number or length of your social activities and excursions as a consequence of your condition. You may find that day-to-day activities the majority of people take for granted become major planning exercises or just impossible. You probably fear feeling embarrassed if others learn of your problem and don't want pity from those closest to you. You may stop visiting with friends because you can't sit still long enough to play one hand of bridge without jumping up to go to the toilet. You're probably uncomfortable at parties and dinners, fretting that an odor of urine surrounds your clothes. Journeys by car or on public transportation are often out of the question, making shopping, visiting places of public interest, entertaining, or socializing almost impossible. Finding accessible public toilets can become a source of major anxiety.

If you wear protective absorbent pads, you probably have the constant fear that urine will leak onto outer garments and furniture. You may find yourself washing underclothes and sheets by hand to hide urine stains from other members of your household. Sleep deprivation is also common, as you probably wake up several times during a night to make trips to the bathroom. You may worry that there won't be a place to change your clothing should you have an accident. You may stop attending church services or going to the movies and the theater. Even long-standing relationships can be broken, sometimes never to be mended again. The consequences of an OAB and incontinence problem can creep into every part of your life.

Avoidance of Travel

Beth's husband just retired and is ready to travel. He wants to go to Europe and tour England, France, and Italy. He has promised this trip to Beth for years. But Beth is worried. She's afraid of going to cities where the bathrooms aren't easily available, and she doesn't think she'll be able to buy her "pads" in Europe. She doesn't know how to explain this to her husband.

Like Beth, if you have OAB, you probably view travel as an insurmountable obstacle. You find yourself making excuses and changes in your daily routine to ensure that traveling to unfamiliar places isn't part of it. When taking a vacation, you try to ensure that your accommodations have appropriate access to a toilet. You may start packing special items when traveling—bedpads, linens, plastic bags, and rubber pants. Vacations and excursions are curtailed, and even short trips away from home are avoided. Grocery shopping is an ordeal because of urgency and frequency, the absence of convenient restrooms, and the worry of getting caught in a long line at the check-out counter. You will go to great lengths to make certain you know where all the bathrooms are located. Travel brings the possibility that there won't be a restroom available when you need one.

OAB, Sex, and Intimacy

Intimacy is a personal and delicate act. The self-image of both sexes is intertwined with sexual performance. Over 50 percent of all sexually active women with incontinence suffer some type of sexual dysfunction. Women report that urinary symptoms adversely affect their sex life because of the fear of urine leakage during intercourse and orgasm. They fear having to interrupt the sex act with the need to urinate. To avoid embarrassment, they avoid intimacy and refrain from discussing the problem with their partner.

Caring for Someone with OAB and Incontinence

Vicky is eighty-three and lives with her sister, Becky. Vicky was diagnosed with Parkinson's Disease several years ago and has rapidly lost her physical functions. She recently moved in with her sister but lately has had increasing problems with urinary urgency and frequency, with occasional urinary incontinence episodes. Becky has adapted well to Vicky's frequent requests to go to the bathroom during the day, but during the night, it's become a great burden. Becky reports waking up four to five times a night to help Vicky to the toilet and is starting to feel the strain.

Do Becky's frustrations sound familiar? You may have a family member like Vicky who has suffered from OAB, and that member is probably a woman. At least 30 percent of the general adult population from every walk of life and in all kinds of physical and mental conditions experience OAB. This requires a health-care system that can handle the needs of people of every social and economic status.

Adults' associate wet underwear with childhood and children. If they develop urine leakage in addition to urgency and frequency, they view it as the beginning of the loss of control over their lives. The possibility of being dependent on others for physical care or the decline of a productive life are difficult situations to face. If such worries become a dominant force in a person's life, some forego prompt and proper care, causing further deterioration in physical and even mental health.

Then, too, Americans are famously obsessed with personal hygiene, and the most often-cited fear of persons with OAB and incontinence is odor. This hygienic fixation contributes to an incontinent person's fear that the smell of urine will cling to them, and maintaining dryness and cleanliness becomes of paramount concern. Some might choose to manage incontinence by themselves by using absorbent products, never investigating less expensive and more effective therapies. Even if a person only has urgency and frequency, they may use absorbent pads on a daily basis "just in case," as the fear of urine leakage is always present. In many cases, this self-management prolongs the problem and creates more complicated problems, extending the course of the condition.

As the aging population increases and home care becomes the norm, family members, especially women who are the primary care givers, need to have knowledge of OAB treatments and how to get help.

Persons at Risk

Overactive bladder may have a specific cause. These causes, or risk factors, affect the anatomy and physiology of the lower urinary tract. Changes or damages to the bladder, urethra, pelvic floor muscles and nerves can result in overactive bladder with incontinence. A neurologic disorder that interferes with the communication between the nerve pathways and the lower urinary tract and pelvic muscles can predispose a person to OAB with or without incontinence.

Age

Getting older doesn't necessarily lead to OAB, although older persons are more vulnerable to developing overactive bladder, most often with incontinence. A study by the Kaiser Health System in San Diego of women seeking treatment for pelvic floor disorders (urinary incontinence, fecal incontinence, and pelvic organ prolapse) showed that most are between forty and eighty years of age, the largest group being between sixty and eighty years of age (Luber 2001). This study also showed that the incidence of overactive bladder and urge incontinence increased with age to greater than 65 percent in patients older than fifty years. Many elderly people have illnesses that will affect their remaining bladder control. The aging process, illness, or trauma can produce changes in the Bladder Control Center in the brain. Neurological changes in the brain stem and spine can produce changes that can give rise to poor coordination of bladder contraction and urinary sphincter opening. Data collected in six European countries showed the prevalence of overactive bladder reaching over 30 percent in men and women older than seventy-five years. Demographic trends in the United States show that the overall population is getting older. By the year 2030, it's projected that the number of women aged sixty years or older will nearly double, compared with only an 8 percent increase in the thirty to fifty-nine age group. Thus, the incidence of OAB can be expected to increase substantially in the next few decades.

Race

Race may be a factor in overactive bladder. OAB with incontinence is felt to be more common in African-American women than in Caucasians, Hispanics, or Asians. Race is a significant risk factor for mixed UI, especially in older African-American women.

Pregnancy and Childbirth

These big physical transitions can cause changes in the lower urinary tract. Urine production increases during pregnancy, with urinary frequency affecting women throughout pregnancy. Both urge and stress incontinence are reported by women during pregnancy, as well as nocturia (getting up frequently at night to urinate). Vaginal delivery and pelvic trauma during childbirth are strongly implicated in the development of persistent SUI. Women who have had even one vaginal birth are more than two-and-a-half times as likely to report UI as those women who have not had children (Viktrup 2001). The prevalence of SUI has been reported to be 30 percent, five years after a first delivery. Half of all women pregnant for the first time experience UI, especially during the last trimester. Incontinence that occurs immediately after childbirth has been associated with use of forceps, vacuum extraction, episiotomy, and pudendal anesthesia during delivery. Vaginal birth, especially when the infant is large or the second stage of labor is protracted, imposes pressure, stretch, and shearing risk to the muscles and nerves of the pelvic floor.

Falls and Fractures

Falling and resulting fractures are relatively common occurrences for older women. Estimates suggest the prevalence of falling to be approximately 30 percent in women living at home who are sixty-five years or older, with an estimated 6 percent of falls resulting in a bone fracture. Falling accounts for the majority of deaths related to injury and is the sixth leading cause of death among older adults. Falling occurs frequently during the night when a person may make frequent attempts to get to the bathroom to urinate (Brown 2000). They will often rush because of urgency and the fear of urine leakage on the way. Surgery to fix a bone fracture from a fall is costly and associated with a considerably increased risk of additional medical complications and death, especially in the frail elderly. A study of women around the age of seventy years showed that urge incontinence was associated with an increased risk of falls and fractures. Women with weekly urge incontinence had a 26 percent increased risk of falling and a 34 percent increased risk of fracture (Brown 2000). With daily urge incontinence, the risks increased to 35 percent for falling and 45 percent for bone fractures (Brown 2000). These findings suggest that early identification and treatment of OAB may have the potential to prevent or decrease falls and bone fractures.

Long-Standing Medical Problems

Chronic medical conditions can contribute to an overactive bladder. During an illness, perception of urgency, the need to urinate, or the sensation of a full bladder can diminish or completely disappear. Recovery from surgery, a serious illness, and bed rest also limit physical mobility and present additional challenges. People who are ill are primarily concerned with their treatment and recovery, and bladder needs are often not clearly or quickly recognized. Response to bladder sensations may be slow or ignored until the urge to void suddenly appears. In many cases, urgency and frequency with subsequent urine leakage is the first indication to an ill person that a bladder problem exists. When the illness resolves, overactive bladder symptoms may or may not resolve. People with heart disease can develop congestive heart failure (CHF) and peripheral venous insufficiency (poor or decreased blood flow to the arms and legs) leading to edema (fluid retention) in the lower part of the legs, ankles, and feet. This can exacerbate urinary frequency, nocturia, and incontinence when the person is lying flat.

Physical Disabilities

These may cause difficulty walking, the inability to use your legs, arms, or your upper or lower body, and impaired hearing or eyesight, all of which can be obstacles to using the toilet. As mentioned above, falling can happen when attempting to urinate. It can be frustrating to face what appears to be an insurmountable obstacle every time a person with a physical disability has to use the bathroom. If you have mobility or balance problems, you may be unable to suppress urgency until a caregiver arrives to help you to the bathroom. Especially for the elderly, physical mobility or limitations present difficulties when using the toilet. They may be unable to walk or propel their wheelchairs to the toilet in a timely fashion. These individuals benefit from convenient bathroom facilities and bedside commodes, sufficient lighting, and special bathroom fixtures such as railings, low toilets, and so on. If toilet facilities are not easily reached and accessible, if a portable bedside commode or urinal is not at hand, or if no one is near to provide assistance in getting up and walking to a bathroom, sitting on a toilet, or using a bedpan, people in this position can grow frustrated. These frustrations can lead to incontinence during some stage of their incapacity. Chronic illnesses (such as rheumatoid arthritis) may restrict movement. Individuals with arthritis may have mobility and dexterity problems, causing a slower and more unsteady gait that can affect the ability to respond to urgency and frequency and limit the ability to get to the toilet safely and in time.

> *Joyce is seventy-four years old and was quite active until she had a stroke. She was always able to control her bladder, but since her stroke she has a difficult time getting up from her chair and she now walks slower. Joyce had two urge incontinent "accidents" yesterday because she just couldn't get to the bathroom quick enough.*

Neurologic Diseases

Diseases of the nervous system can affect the bladder by interrupting the messages that usually get sent to the bladder. Angie's story provides a good illustration.

> *Angie is forty-six years old and was diagnosed with multiple sclerosis ten years ago. Angie is worried that her husband will leave her if he learns about her accidents, both bladder and bowel. Angie will feel humiliated if he finds out; he's been able to handle the MS, but Angie isn't sure he could handle this. Angie's problem with bladder and bowel management has to do with urgency rather than full incontinence. She must make a daily plan to allow for quick and easy availability of an accessible bathroom. Angie has become somewhat physically disabled and needs to use a wheelchair, and it takes more time for her to transfer from a chair or scooter to a commode. Angie feels she's become obsessed with her disease and her needs.*

The following are examples of neurologic conditions that may lead to symptoms of OAB.

Multiple sclerosis (MS) is a chronic disease of the nervous system characterized by fluctuating loss of coordination and strength of muscles, as well as bladder problems. With MS, spinal-cord lesions interrupt the nerve pathways from the brain to the lower spinal cord, causing bladder overactivity. Difficulty with urination occurs in about 80 percent of people who have MS. The loss of bladder control may be temporary, improving as the symptoms of the disease improves. However, most persons with MS live with persistent urinary frequency and incontinence.

Parkinson's disease (PD) is a degenerative disease of the nervous system characterized by tremor, rigidity, and bladder dysfunction. Muscle weakness affects the sphincter muscles, causing both urinary and fecal incontinence. OAB with frequency and urgency are common urinary symptoms in PD, with the prevalence of urinary symptoms in persons diagnosed with PD reported to be between 37 to 71 percent. Rigidity of muscles contributes to the inability to get to the toilet.

Cerebrovascular Accident (CVA) or "stroke" can lead to bladder dysfunction. A stroke occurs when a blood vessel that feeds the brain gets clogged or bursts. The affected part of the brain can't work, and neither can the part of the body it controls. Stroke frequency increases with advancing age. Men are more likely to have strokes than woman, and African-Americans are more likely to have strokes than Caucasians. OAB, incontinence, and other bladder dysfunction can occur after a stroke, usually within the first few days. Many individuals experience a lack of sensory awareness to urinate or an inability to control their bladder emptying. Depending on the severity of the stroke and its affect on speech, many stroke victims may be unable to communicate their toileting needs. Common bladder symptoms include frequency and urgency, and urinary retention may also cause overflow incontinence. A common bladder condition that occurs after a stroke is often referred to as *uninhibited neurogenic bladder dysfunction*. This is when a person is able to sense the need to urinate and can start the stream, but cannot delay urination. Often the urge sensation is perceived when only small amounts of urine are present in the bladder.

Diabetes can lead to common urinary symptoms, frequency and urgency, incomplete bladder emptying, and urinary tract infections. If you have diabetes you have a 30 to 70 percent increased risk of developing urge incontinence. As the diabetes progresses, you may develop nerve damage or neuropathy (a disorder that affects the nervous system), which can lead to urinary retention. People with nerve damage as a result of diabetes have a reduced sensation to urinate. Causes of OAB and incontinence are not well understood in people who have Diabetes. Poorly controlled blood sugars in diabetes may cause increased urine volume and frequency. Diabetes may cause nerve damage to the bladder muscle leading to loss of muscle function and the inability to control urinating. Finally, diabetes increases your chance of developing UTIs.

Medications

Bladder sensation can be reduced by medications, especially if you're taking more than one. Any drug that alters, slows, or dulls the nerves or brain can affect your bladder. Also, many older adults with chronic illnesses are prescribed multiple medications that contribute to or in many cases cause overactive bladder. For example, if you have pain and take a pain medication, the urge sensation or message sent by the brain telling you to urinate may be diminished or delayed. Many drug references or books list the OAB symptoms of urgency and frequency as possible side effects of hundreds, if not thousands, of registered drugs currently on the market. Overactive bladder among the elderly is often caused by prescribed drugs and often is overlooked by the doctors prescribing them. The more drugs you take, the greater the chance of side effects, including loss of bladder control. The following are common medications taken by older adults that put them at risk for OAB and incontinence:

♦ **Diuretics** or "water pills" take excess water out of the bloodstream by increasing the amount of urine volume. People taking HCTZ (Hydrochlorothiazide or Dyazide), furosemide (Lasix), and bumetanide (Bumex) may not have time to get to the bathroom before they leak. The time of day you take your water pill is important. If a person is urinating several times during the night, taking the pill in the early or mid-afternoon may help.

♦ **Sedatives, antidepressants, and pain killers** dull the senses and may decrease your sensation of the need to urinate. If you take a sleeping pill, it's unlikely that you'll be conscious enough to receive the message to go to the bathroom when your bladder is full. Sleeping pills and sedatives can cause an artificially deep sleep, masking urinary urgency. Also, they can make you feel groggy and disoriented on the way to the bathroom, increasing the chances of falling. The bladder will not get the urge message in time for the person to get safely to the bathroom. Confusion and disorientation is also a side effect of sedatives and the person may not be alert enough to recognize the bladder's needs. These medications may also cause decreased bladder contractions, leading to incomplete bladder emptying.

◆ **Narcotics or painkillers** deprive a person of clear sensory perception. A person will not sense or feel the need to urinate. If the person becomes constipated while using narcotics (a common side effect), excessive pressure is exerted on the bladder by the hard stool, decreasing its ability to hold urine and increasing urgency.

◆ **Alcohol** has a sedative effect that may affect a person's urge sensation or the awareness of the need to urinate. At the same time, alcohol's diuretic effect causes the body to produce a larger volume of urine that the person may not be able to accommodate causing incontinence.

Low Fluid Intake

If you don't take in enough fluid during the day, your urine can become highly concentrated, leading to irritation of your bladder and urethra and resulting in urinary frequency or incontinence. Maintaining adequate fluid intake is important, especially for older adults who already have a decrease in total body water and are at risk for dehydration. Some people mistakenly believe that not drinking water and other beverages several hours before traveling will decrease the chances of urgency and frequency. In certain cases, drinking the recommended amount of eight eight-ounce glasses of water per day may eliminate bothersome urgency.

Pelvic-Muscle Weakness

Weak pelvic floor muscles in women can be due to loss of nerve fibers related to childbirth and often leads to OAB. Prolapse (sagging or dropping) of the pelvic organs from a weak pelvic muscle can cause poor pelvic support of the bladder and urethra, resulting in their lying below their normal positions, leading to defects in the transmission of pressures to the sphincter area. When the muscles of the pelvic floor are weak or lax, even if they're not fully prolapsed, the portion of the urethra closest to the bladder tends to lie below the pelvic floor. This can lead to a feeling of pressure and urinary urgency. With a rise in the bladder pressure and pelvic-muscle relaxation, stress incontinence can also occur.

Depression

This difficult emotional condition often goes hand in hand with urge urinary incontinence. Adult women with bladder-control problems indicate more anxiety and emotional distress than continent adults and more than in persons with other types of incontinence (Dugan 2001). Many incontinent persons become depressed and, in time, develop severe psychological and physiological problems. The association between depression and urinary symptoms may be related to altered neurotransmitters (chemicals, like serotonin, that help transmit messages from the brain) in the lower spinal cord.

Environmental Barriers

Obstacles in the environment and in your living environment may contribute to your overactive bladder problems. Poor bathroom accessibility, hazards confronting you on the way to the toilet, and inadequate toilet facilities can negatively impact you if you have OAB. By observing how you use the bathroom facilities, a medical provider can suggest ways to help you reduce the time it takes to use the toilet. When this toilet time is reduced, you may regain your bladder control. Equipment that enhances mobility such as canes, walkers, and wheelchairs should be available if you have problems walking. OAB can occur if you're unable to reach the bathroom because of obstacles such as furniture or other objects, poor lighting, or the need to climb stairs. The presence of a commode chair, bathroom grab bars, raised toilet-seat, and toilet seat arms make your home more "user friendly." In some cases it is helpful if toilets are at least seventeen inches high, with arms to assist you in lowering to or rising from the toilet seat. Wheelchair patients find themselves in a special bind. Bathrooms in older homes and nursing homes and restroom facilities located in public buildings that were built before the American with Disabilities Act (ADA) was enacted are not always equipped to handle wheelchairs. Even though ADA mandates that entrances, exits, and restrooms must be handicapped accessible, many bathrooms and restrooms are still reachable only by stairs, which, of course, can't be climbed when you're in a wheel chair. Wheelchair-bound individuals must be taught an easy method for using the toilet. If you're confined to a bed, male and female urinals, bedside commodes, or bedpans (sometimes called collective devices), can all help maintain continence.

There are other, more personal environmental factors. Clothing is, at times, a barrier to toilet use. The number of clothes or pads you wear to protect yourself from urine leakage can actually hinder bathroom use. It can be very hard for arthritic fingers to unzip or unbutton pants. Assessing your coordination and ability to lift up and pull down your clothes is essential. Adjusting clothing to make disrobing easier can reduce your bathroom discomfit. You should choose clothing that is easy to remove in the bathroom—wide, lift-up skirts, lapover skirts, and elastic or tie pants. As a rule, replace buttons at the waist with Velcro strips or snap enclosures. In addition to clothing, simply getting to a bathroom can become a problem for those with OAB. Families, nursing homes, and public facilities must ensure that their bathroom and restroom facilities are conveniently located. Proper design should result in easy access and use.

Menopause, Lack of Estrogen, and OAB

Joellis stopped menstruating four months ago and since then has noticed problems with urinary urgency. She feels like she always has to go to the bathroom. Sex with her husband is uncomfortable because her vagina feels so dry. When she visited her nurse practitioner for her yearly pap smear, the nurse mentioned that Joellis' vaginal tissue had become, thinner and recommended an estrogen-based cream to keep the vaginal tissues moist and to keep the muscles toned. The estrogen would help the tissue of her bladder and urethra stay strong and supple. Once Joellis started using the cream, her problems with urinary urgency and frequent urination decreased.

After menopause, a woman's level of the hormone estrogen lowers dramatically. This is a problem, as without sufficient estrogen, the tissues of the vagina and urethra become thinner, drier, and may be more susceptible to irritation. This deficiency weakens the pelvic-floor tissue and urethra, a condition called *urogenital atrophy* or *atrophic vaginitis*. The area around the woman's vagina and urethra can become inflamed, causing frequency and urgency that can precipitate incontinence. Vaginal dryness is commonly the first reported symptom of the condition. Painful and difficult urination, burning sensations in the vaginal area, itching, frequent urination, painful intercourse, and urinary incontinence are indications of vaginitis. Symptoms may not develop until several years after menopause when levels of estrogen in the tissue fall below the levels needed to support cell growth. Use of an estrogen preparation such as a cream, tablet, or ring placed in the vagina may improve these symptoms. These preparations are low doses of estrogen and will not cause many of the side effects that are seen in oral estrogen replacement treatment. Because of the recent report that has appeared about the risks (and benefits) of estrogen treatment, a health-care provider should always be involved in the decision for such treatment and decide upon the preparation, dose, and length of use (Lacey, et al. 2002).

Overweight and OAB Symptoms

Being overweight can contribute to OAB. Even a few pounds can make a difference. The OAB symptoms seen in obesity may be secondary to increased pressure on the bladder and greater abnormal movement of the urethra. Also, obesity may impair blood flow or nerve innervation to the bladder. A 5 to 10 percent weight loss can significantly reduce the intra-abdominal pressure that puts added stress or pressure on your bladder, causing leakage of small amounts of urine. If you think your weight may be contributing to your OAB, consider losing a few pounds and see if your symptoms improve.

Smoking and OAB

Smoking increases the risk of developing all forms of UI, and stress UI in particular, depending on the number of cigarettes smoked. It is felt that smoker's cough (more violent and frequent than non-smoker's coughs) promotes the earlier development of stress UI. There may also be an association between nicotine and increased detrusor contractions.

If you thought that OAB is only about the bladder, we have a surprise for you. Your bowels can have a significant impact on your bladder—how it stores and empties urine. The next chapter discusses the interrelationship between your bladder and your bowels and provides remedies for maintaining bowel regularity.

Chapter 5

The Relationship Between Bowel Disorders and OAB

Mike is seventy-nine and used to take several different laxatives every day. When he was young and active, his bowels were regular, working every day like clockwork. Once he stopped jogging five years ago, he noticed a change. If his bowels didn't move for two days, he would take Milk of Magnesia. If that didn't work, he took Dulcolax tablets and sometimes even mineral oil. He would sometimes go five days without having a bowel movement, and then his wife had to give him an enema. Mike felt that when his bowels weren't working, his bladder was overworking. He began noticing that when he didn't move his bowels, he had more urinary urgency and frequency. When he mentioned this to his doctor, he suggested that Mike see a nurse practitioner who specializes in both bladder and bowel problems. The nurse practitioner gave Mike a bowel schedule. He was told to sit on the toilet every morning after breakfast, since food (especially warm food and drink) stimulate the bowels to move. Mike was to raise his feet on a footstool when he sat on the toilet because this position aids in bowel evacuation. If his stool is hard, Mike was told to put a glycerin suppository in his rectum. Mike was also told to take a special bran recipe. After three weeks of following these instructions, Mike saw a big difference. He was having a bowel movement almost every day on schedule after breakfast. He didn't need anymore enemas, and he noticed that as his bowel movements became regular, his OAB symptoms improved.

Mike was right in realizing that control of his bladder is linked to his bowels, since the regularity or irregularity of bowel movements impacts your bladder and its ability to empty. Many people with OAB may experience constipation and/or fecal (bowel) incontinence. The reason both bladder and bowel problems may occur at the same time is that the digestive tract and the lower urinary tract are closely connected, and anything that affects one of them can affect the other. These systems share common nerves and are supported by the pelvic muscles that play a vital role in maintaining bowel and bladder control. As we mentioned in chapter 2, the urinary tract and the digestive tract get their nerves from a common source, the pudendal nerve. Therefore, anything that cuts or damages this source of nerve supply can cause OAB and bowel dysfunction. Diseases or injuries that affect the spinal cord or the nerves or muscles in this area can affect both systems. This chapter reviews the causes of these bowel disorders and provides you with practical solutions for maintaining or regaining bowel regularity.

Understanding How the Bowels Function

The intestine consists of the small and large intestine. The large intestine or colon is a hollow muscular tube about five feet in length and plays a significant part in normal bowel function. It is divided into the cecum, colon, and rectum. The *cecum* comprises the first two or three inches of the large intestine. The *colon* is subdivided into the ascending, transverse, descending, and sigmoid colon (see Figure 5). The last portion of the large intestine is the *rectum,* which extends from the sigmoid colon to the anus (about six inches). The last inch of the rectum is called the anal canal. It contains the internal and external anal sphincters, which play an important role in regulating defecation (having a bowel movement). Muscle contractions in the colon push the stool toward the anus. By the time it reaches the rectum, it is solid, because most of the water has been absorbed. The large intestine has many functions, all related to the final processing of intestinal contents. Very little, if any, digestion takes place in the large intestine, the most important function of which is the absorption of water and electrolytes. Approximately twenty ounces of water is absorbed daily from the intestinal contents. The longer the fecal mass stays in the colon, the more water is absorbed.

Movement of the intestinal contents through the large intestine is called *peristalsis* and is usually slow. *Mass peristalsis,* which is a

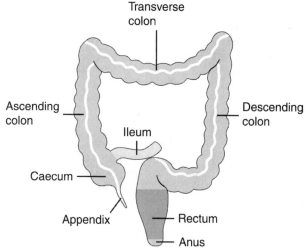

Figure 5: The Large Bowel

contraction involving a large segment of the colon, moves the feces (stool) mass into the sigmoid colon where it is stored. This occurs two to three times per day, especially after breakfast. The external anal sphincter is controlled by the pudendal nerve, the same nerve that controls the external urinary sphincter. Like the urinary tract, the nerve supply to the large intestine contains both parasympathetic and sympathetic nerves. In general, stimulation of the sympathetic fibers inhibits activity in the intestinal tract. It also excites the internal anal sphincter. Stimulation of the parasympathetic fibers causes an increase in bowel activity and in the defecation reflexes.

Having a Bowel Movement

Defecation is a reflex involving the muscles of the anal canal and end of the rectum. Entry of the feces into the rectum distends the rectal walls and stimulates mass peristaltic movements of the bowel, which moves the feces toward the anus. As the stool nears the anus, the internal anal sphincter is inhibited and if the external anal sphincter is relaxed (under voluntary control), defecation will occur. The defecation reflex may be halted by voluntary contraction of the external anal sphincter. When this is done, the defecation reflex dies out after a few minutes and usually won't return for several hours. Water continues to be absorbed from the fecal mass, causing it to become firmer so that subsequent defecation is more difficult. If this pattern continues, you may be faced with constipation. Defecation may be made easier by an increase in intra-abdominal pressure brought about by simultaneous contraction of the chest muscles and abdominal muscles (called Valsalva's maneuver or straining).

Constipation and OAB

Constipation is a bowel problem that is more common than people believe. It's usually defined as the infrequent and difficult passage of stool with fewer than three bowel movements per week. If more than three days pass without a bowel movement, your intestinal contents, called stool or feces, may harden or become pellet-like. You may have difficulty or even pain when having a bowel movement and use excessive straining to pass the stool. Constipation and lower urinary tract symptoms (called LUTS) such as those seen in persons with OAB very frequently occur in the elderly, and dysfunction in either of these systems may affect the other. Older adults are 5 times more likely than younger adults to report problems with constipation. Many people, especially as they age, tend to be "bowel obsessive." Every year, Americans spend millions of dollars on laxatives and drugs to make their bowels move. Many times, older adults become overly concerned with having a daily bowel movement and constipation may be imaginary. If you also have urinary urgency, frequency, and incontinence, you often see improvement in these OAB symptoms once constipation is resolved.

What is a Normal Bowel Movement?

Many people have misconceptions concerning normal bowel habits. You may feel that a bowel movement is necessary every day. It's important to understand that bowel patterns vary and that having a bowel movement every other day or three times a week may be normal. Also, you may feel that the longer feces sit in your colon, the more "toxins" your body absorbs. Therefore, you may find yourself taking large amounts and many different types of laxatives to have daily bowel movements that will get rid of "harmful wastes." Heavy dependence on laxatives can become habit-forming. Routine use of laxatives can interfere with your bowels so that, over time, your bowels have an even more difficult time moving. Plenty of other problems come with habitual use of laxatives, so you should only use them occasionally.

There are several factors that can prevent you from having a regular, normal bowel movement and they are listed as follows:

- **Unbalanced diet,** especially diets high in animal fats and refined sugars, tend to be low in fiber. Low-fiber diets result in less frequent bowel movements and more problems with constipation.

- **Poor or low intake of water** and other fluids cause bowel movements to be hard, less frequent, and harder to pass.

- **Laxative abuse** can contribute to long term bowel dysfunction (especially if you habitually take laxatives). You can become dependent upon them and may require increasing dosages to get the effects you want. But eventually your intestine will become accustomed to the laxatives and won't respond to them properly. Also, long-term use of laxatives can cause electrolyte abnormalities.

- **Change in your normal routine,** especially travel, can interfere with your bowel pattern, especially if travel consists of long-distance trips and trips to other countries. This may be due to changes in drinking water, schedule, diet, and a lack of exercise.

- **Hemorrhoids** are swollen veins in the anus or rectum that are often a result of constipation. They can be internal, inside the rectum or external, outside the anal opening. Hemorrhoids can cause pain, itching, and discomfort when a person has a bowel movement and cause spasms of the anal sphincter delaying bowel movements.

- **Medications** commonly prescribed for older adults cause constipation. This is especially true with pain medications, antidepressants, antacids that contain aluminum, iron supplements, and tranquilizers.

- **Diseases** such as multiple sclerosis, Parkinson's, and occurrences such as stroke or spinal cord injury affect nerves leading to the intestines, rectum, and anus and can cause constipation. As mentioned in chapter 4, these are some of the same diseases that also contribute to OAB.

- **Pregnancy** often leads to problems with constipation. The reason may be due to increased pressure from the baby on the intestines or hormonal changes.

♦ **Lack of exercise** or prolonged bed rest due to an accident or illness may contribute to constipation.

Bowel or Fecal Incontinence

Bowel or fecal incontinence is the involuntary loss of liquid, solid stool, or gas from the anus at inappropriate times. If you have this problem, you may find yourself evacuating your bowels into your clothing without any warning. Having both urinary and bowel (fecal) incontinence is so difficult to manage that sufferers live in a constant state of anxiety and may totally withdraw from society. In women, the most common cause of fecal incontinence is trauma to the pelvic and rectal area from childbirth or surgery, usually causing an injury to either the anal sphincter or the pudendal nerves. Rectal sensation warnings or the urgency of imminent defecation helps you discriminate between formed and unformed stool and gas. Impaired rectal sensation may deprive you of this useful information and result in fecal incontinence.

Among older adults, the most common cause of fecal incontinence is neither loss of mobility nor dementia but simply the natural effects of aging on the body. Muscles and tissues weaken, lose their elasticity, and become lax. Changes in muscle strength, muscle mass, and muscle and nerve reflexes affect the rectal area just as they affect your arms and legs. Thus, some older adults can't retain gas or stool, especially liquid stool, for as long as they once could. Also, an older adult may not be able to reflexively close the anal sphincter quickly enough to avoid a fecal accident. If you have fecal incontinence, you may have less rectal sensation and less sphincter strength than people who do not have fecal incontinence. Severe constipation can lead to bowel incontinence. Also, constipation can lead to a large amount of stool in the rectum, which can lead to fecal impaction.

Normalizing Your Bowel Movements

To maintain good bowel control and to prevent bowel dysfunction and related OAB, you need to keep a normal routine for having bowel movements. We would like to give you some suggestions that we've recommended to many of our patients. We believe that dietary and lifestyle improvements can lessen the chances of constipation and other bowel problems.

Fluids

Drinking plenty of fluids, preferably water, helps stimulate intestinal activity. Drink at least six to eight eight-ounce glasses of caffeine-free liquids per day. Fluids aid the passage of bowel movements and also help prevent dehydration. Prune juice has almost no fiber, but does have a laxative effect, probably because of its content of magnesium salts. Apricot juice has high fiber content.

Fiber

Foods rich in fiber can help you avoid constipation by adding bulk to the stool, allowing an easier movement. If you have constipation, you should increase your dietary fiber to twenty to thirty grams per day. High-fiber foods include:

♦ Whole grain bread contains 8 to 10 percent dietary fiber, but some fiber-rich breakfast cereals (like All-Bran) contain 25 percent.

♦ Raw vegetables, especially green leafy ones, and fresh fruits with skins (like apples) are good fiber options. Vegetables contain cellulose, hemicellulose, and lignin. Lignin is not digested in the human intestine and, therefore, adds to stool weight. Prunes are relatively high in fiber (two grams).

♦ Wild and brown rice are rich in fiber content.

A solution to constipation, if you can tolerate wheat products, is to use whole, unprocessed, coarse wheat bran, often called Miller's bran. This is not the same type of bran that's in the widely advertised commercial bran cereals. Whole, unprocessed, coarse bran is natural and a person cannot take too much of it. Miller's bran can be purchased very inexpensively at health-food stores and local grocery stores. This form of bran does not dissolve in liquids, so you should consider sprinkling it on breakfast cereal and develop a routine of adding one or two tablespoons to foods such as yogurt, Jell-O, cottage cheese, ice cream, or puddings. When cooking, put bran in sauces, muffins, gravies, and soups.

It's best to start with small quantities and work your way up. Begin with one tablespoon of bran, and gradually, over time, increase the amount. A common and successful recipe is mixing together:

1 cup applesauce
1 cup coarse, unprocessed wheat bran
¾ cup prune juice

Take two tablespoons of the mixture every day, eating it in the evening for a morning bowel movement. Increase the bran mixture by one tablespoon until your bowel movements become regular. If the amount exceeds four tablespoons, take the mixture in divided doses in the morning and evening. Always drink one large glass of water with the mixture. Another bran mixture called "Power Pudding" can also be successful and includes mixing and blending the following ingredients:

½ cup prune juice
½ cup applesauce
½ cup wheat bran flakes
 cup whipped topping
½ cup stewed prunes (canned)

Take ¼ cup portions of the Power Pudding recipe with breakfast and regulate the amount as needed. You can keep the mixture for one week. Additional remedies includes this mixture:

1 lb raisins
1 lb currants
1 lb prunes
1 lb figs
1 lb dates
One (1) 28-ounce container of undiluted prune concentrate.

Put the fruit through a blender and mix with prune concentrate in large mixer (the mixture will be very thick.) Store in a large-mouthed plastic container. All of these mixtures should be covered and stored in a refrigerator. Start by eating two tablespoons of this mixture every morning at breakfast time. Add one tablespoon at at a time until you have a soft stool.

Use of bran can have side effects including increased flatulence (gas), abdominal bloating, and cramps but, by starting out small and increasing the amount slowly, side effects can be avoided. In any case, if they do occur, they'll disappear in a few weeks.

Movement

Some form of daily exercise helps your bowels to stay regular.

Routine

It's helpful to begin a routine bowel-movement schedule. Sufficient time should be set aside to allow for undisturbed visits to the bathroom. The optimal time is in the morning, after breakfast. Both eating and the smell of appetizing foods can cause the bowels to move. Drink something warm with your breakfast, such as warm water, as this will help the bowels to move. In addition, never ignore the urge to have a bowel movement. This is especially important for residents in a nursing home who need assistance to the toilet. If a regular toileting time is not set aside for the resident to empty their bowels, they will likely have bowel "accidents." Try to avoid using a bedpan, if at all possible, if you are or are caring for a bedridden person who may be living at home or in a nursing home. Using a bedpan in the prone (lying flat and on your back) position can cause undue strain if the person is not properly positioned. It forces the extension of legs, pushes the stomach (abdomen) out, and does not allow muscles to aid in defecation. Gravity and sitting upright assists in the passage of stool, so putting your feet up on a footstool and pushing your body slightly forward while on the toilet can aid in moving your bowels. Massaging or rubbing the lower part of your stomach to push the bowel movement into the rectum is also helpful. Also remember that it may take some time, about twenty to thirty minutes, to have a bowel movement.

Suppositaries

Inserting a suppository into the rectum (like glycerine or Dulcolax) can make it easier to move the bowels. Insert the suppository about fifteen minutes after a meal, preferably breakfast. Use daily until a consistent bowel pattern is identified. Digital stimulation, which is putting a lubricated (with K-Y Jelly) finger in the rectum, can also help your bowels to move.

Laxatives

There are certain laxatives that can help your constipation. The most common laxatives used for bowel dysfunction, especially constipation are the following:

- ♦ Stool softeners (like Colace and Pericolace) provide moisture to the stool and prevent excessive loss of water. They are often recommended after surgery and childbirth. They work within twenty-four to forty-eight hours and produce a firm, semisolid stool.

♦ Lubricants (like mineral oil) grease the stool, allowing it to slip through the intestine more easily. You should feel the effects within six to eight hours. Mineral oil can block the absorption of vitamins A,D,E, and K and may also interact with other drugs, therefore, it should be taken with care.

♦ Bulk-forming laxatives (like FiberCon, Metamucil, and Citrucel) are the safest laxatives, but they can interfere with absorption of some drugs. They should be taken with eight ounces of water, since they absorb water in the intestine to make your stool softer. These types of laxatives can take twelve hours to three days to work.

♦ Osmotic cathartics (like Milk of Magnesia, Miralax, and Lactulose) work by causing water to remain in the intestine for easier movement of stool. They produce watery stool in three to six hours and can be helpful for severe constipation. Milk of Magnesia pushes stool through the intestines so fast that nutrients are not completely absorbed, so do not exceed recommended doses.

♦ Stimulant laxatives (like Senna, Senekot, Dulcolax, Correctol, and Ex-lax) that increase bowel peristalsis by altering the exchange of electrolytes in the intestinal wall should only be used occasionally, since they can cause dependency and can damage your bowels with continual use and often can cause diarrhea. Effects are usually noted within six to eight hours.

♦ Enemas (like tap water, saline, Fleets, Milk & Molasses) instill fluid into the rectum for removal of stool. But don't use enemas often, because they can lead to a loss of normal bowel function and cause decreased rectal tone.

♦ Suppositories (like glycerine, Dulcolax) trigger the defecation reflex and cause the rectum to empty any stool contents. They work within fifteen minutes.

Now that you know about the relationship between your bladder and bowels, you need to learn more about your individual OAB problem. You may need to seek some professional advice, but before you seek a medical provider, it's important to keep a voiding diary to determine the extent of your OAB problem.

Chapter 6

When To Seek Help

The time to seek help for your OAB is when symptoms first occur, and the first line of defense is finding a competent medical provider. If they can't help solve your problem, they'll refer you to a specialist. Writing down your symptoms, problems, and questions before visiting a medical provider is a good idea. This allows you to think about your problem before your visit. Answering the most commonly asked questions before seeing a medical provider allows you more time to think about your answers so that you thoroughly understand your OAB and can explain it effectively. We have listed questions we usually ask our patients.

1. Do you ever leak urine when you don't want to?

2. Do you have strong, sudden urges to urinate that are difficult to control?

3. Do you lose urine on your way to the bathroom?

4. Do you often go to the bathroom more than eight times during the day?

5. Do you awaken at night to urinate? If yes, how many times?

6. Do you always go to the bathroom when you're near one, just in case, or because you're afraid of wetting yourself?

7. When you're in a new place, do you make sure you know the location of the restroom?

8. Do you frequently limit your fluid intake when you're away from home so that you won't have to worry about finding a restroom?

9. Are you reluctant to take a vacation, go for car rides, or travel because you fear that you won't be able to find a restroom when you need it?

10. Do you experience an urge to urinate when you see or hear the sound of running water?

11. Do you use pads or diapers to protect your clothes from wetting?

If you have answered "yes" to any of these questions you probably have OAB.

There are additional questions that relate to other common bladder disorders. You should consider these questions also.

1. Do you lose or leak urine when you laugh, cough, sneeze, or lift heavy objects? (Stress Urinary Incontinence)

2. Do you leak urine when you exercise? Have you had to switch or stop doing your sport of choice because you leaked urine? (Stress Incontinence)

3. Do you dribble urine after you urinate? (Overflow)

4. Do you wake up from sleep wet? (Functional)

5. Have you lost urine during or after sex? During your menses? During pregnancy or after childbirth? At the onset of menopause? (Stress Incontinence)

6. Do you have difficulty starting your urine flow? (Overflow)

Now that you have answered important questions about your OAB, you need to track your symptoms by using a record called a "Bladder Diary."

The Importance of a Bladder Diary

As part of determining the specifics of your OAB, your medical provider will need a "picture" of your problem. You can provide this picture by keeping a Bladder Diary or Bladder Record. Most of us don't pay much attention to the number of times we urinate during the day. We've developed comfortable urinary patterns and only when we're forced to deviate from usual patterns is our awareness heightened. Special circumstances—the unavailability of a restroom, an illness, or a persistent bladder condition—abruptly turn our attention to the needs of our bladder. A Bladder Diary is a good way to help identify your condition and symptoms and plan a course of action to control your problem. A diary is a written record of these events and illustrates what happens with your bladder during the course of your day and night. Keep a Bladder Diary for three to five days if you:

♦ Have suddenly started having urinary urgency

♦ Find yourself going to the bathroom more frequently than usual

♦ Start experiencing "urinary accidents"

♦ Can't determine why your urine leakage or "accidents" have begun

Based on the urinary patterns you record, you and your medical provider can begin to design a plan of action. Consider Estelle's story.

Estelle is a fifty-two-year-old administrative assistant to a company executive who works from 7AM to late in the evening. For years, Estelle has been stopping by the bathroom to urinate before she goes to work, once she arrives at work, before most meetings, and before and after lunch. It seems like she is in the bathroom more often than at her desk. Since she usually gets home after 7PM, she has a late dinner and finds herself getting up two to three times to urinate during the night. Lately, Estelle has to really rush to make it to the bathroom in time, and this is bothering her. She feels that she should mention it to her doctor.

A Bladder Diary would help Estelle pinpoint the presence of urgency, urinary frequency, and any pattern of incontinence episodes, as well as daily fluid intake. The correlation between voiding patterns, severity of urinary urgency, frequency, and urine leakage helps a medical provider determine your baseline urinary patterns. Keeping a written diary concentrates attention on the Bladder Control Center messages sent out by the brain to your bladder telling you to urinate. The diary also gives clues, both to you and your medical provider, as to the effect OAB has on your social life, personal hygiene, and your lifestyle in general. You should record information in your diary throughout the day. This doesn't end when you go to bed, as it's important to understand what you're doing at night. Some OAB experts feel that keeping a Bladder Diary is actually a form of therapy, as you may find that when you start to see habits that are contributing to your OAB, you can modify your behavior, thus decreasing symptoms.

Estelle's doctor asked her to keep a Bladder Diary for three days. At first she thought it was a nuisance, but by the second day she started to notice that she was going to the bathroom every hour, especially when she was at work. She also saw that she was drinking a lot of coffee and tea. She was surprised at the amount of soda and water she was drinking after dinner, and she decided to cut back on the soda.

Estelle was able to notice corollary patterns to her behavior and urination. If you have OAB, you can benefit from completing a Bladder Diary, so let's review how to do one.

How to Complete Your Bladder Diary

This chapter contains a blank Bladder Diary for you to copy and use to record your bladder patterns. As an urologist and nurse practitioner who specialize in bladder conditions such as OAB, we have found this Bladder Diary to be extremely important in providing us with the information we need to make the right decision about each individual's condition. Each column requests specific information that provides a picture of your individual symptoms and is described below.

Column 1

Place a check or an "X" next to the time you go to the bathroom and urinate in the toilet during the day or night. For example, some people get up frequently during the night to urinate. Others may go to the bathroom every time they hear running water. It is important that you mark each time you urinate, even if the amount of urine voided is small.

Column 2

Note the degree or severity of urgency associated with your need to urinate. This is an important OAB symptom, and understanding how bothersome your urgency is will help in your treatment process. We recommend you use the following scale when rating your urgency:

0 = No urgency or need to use the toilet.

1 = Moderate means that the urgency is *tolerated or controlled,* and you can continue with your usual activity for a short time.

2 = Severe is when the urgency is causing extreme difficulty and you *need to stop all of your activity to urinate.*

Column 3

Note each time you leak urine or have accidents (accidental leakage of urine). Use the following code to indicate the amount of urine:

Small = slightly damp or drops.

Moderate = pad or underwear definitely wet, at least a tablespoon

Large = wet outer garments, large urine loss.

If you wear pads, it may be difficult to know how much you leak. Under this circumstance, note either a small amount or a large amount (one that causes you to have to change your pad, diaper, or adult briefs).

Column 4

Describe the activity you were doing when the accident occurred such as getting to the bathroom, laughing, or lifting a heavy object. You should also record any important factors regarding each incident. This helps you and your medical provider determine the causes of the incident.

Column 5

Note the time and type of liquid intake (like coffee, water, etc.) and estimate the amount (for instance, one cup) you drank. Many people falsely believe that by drinking fewer liquids, they will cut down on incidents of urgency, frequency, and urine leakage.

At the bottom of the Bladder Diary are pictures of commercially available products. If you have OAB and experience urine leakage, you may be using tissue or homemade products or commercial protection known as incontinence absorbent products. We ask our patients to circle the products they are using and provide us with the number of products they use each day. As the different products have different absorbency, understanding the type and number of products give us an understanding of the degree of your incontinence.

Once you have recorded your urinating patterns for several days by keeping a Diary, you may need to seek the help of a medical provider who can suggest solutions to your OAB.

Bladder Diary

Date: _____

Time	Voided (X) in Toilet	Circle Degree of Urgency	Urine Leakage	Activity when Leakage Occurred	Liquid Intake
6–8AM		0 1 2	S M L		
8–10AM		0 1 2	S M L		
10AM–12PM		0 1 2	S M L		
12–2PM		0 1 2	S M L		
2–4PM		0 1 2	S M L		
4–6PM		0 1 2	S M L		
6–8PM		0 1 2	S M L		
8–10PM		0 1 2	S M L		
10PM–12AM		0 1 2	S M L		
12–2AM		0 1 2	S M L		
2–4AM		0 1 2	S M L		
4–6AM		0 1 2	S M L		

These are pictures of the most commonly used incontinence products. Circle the product you are using and the number of products you use each day _____.

Pantyliner

Pads or Guards

Undergarment

Protective Underwear

Briefs

If you are not using any of these products tell us what you are using:

☐ Nothing   ☐ Tissue   ☐ Homemade _____

Chapter 7

Investigating the Cause of OAB

An objective determination of your OAB is the first and most important part of the evaluation and treatment process. Symptoms of bladder and urinary tract problems may indicate the presence of OAB, but again, they may not. Neither do they always provide clues as to the possible cause of your problem. That is why the assessment of OAB should be performed by a competent medical provider who understands causes and treatments for OAB.

Choosing Your Medical Provider

There are several types of medical providers who are qualified to assess your OAB. The different types of medical providers are described below.

Physicians

Most persons have a unique relationship with their family doctor, who is usually a general practitioner or an internist and may be called your "primary care physician." A family doctor maintains your medical history—a record of illnesses, medication use, tests, and surgeries. In many cases, after a discussion of symptoms, an examination, and possibly some tests, your family doctor will design a treatment plan for specific symptoms. However, if you have more complex conditions such as cancer, an enlarged prostate, or repeated urinary tract infections, your family doctor will usually refer you to a specialist. There are several different types of specialists who you may see for OAB.

Urologists

The urologist is the physician who is most familiar with OAB and incontinence, as they specialize in all conditions of the urinary tract. Some urologists specialize in primarily treating women with bladder and pelvic-floor conditions.

Gynecologists

For women, a group of doctors called gynecologists treat conditions of the urinary and reproductive systems. Traditionally, they've been the primary physician in dealing with problems arising from pelvic organs. During your yearly gynecologic exam, the gynecologist should ask you if you have any bladder control or urinary symptoms that interfere with your daily routines or lifestyle. A relatively new specialist, the urogynecologist, has emerged from this group. They are gynecologists who have additional training in bladder disorders.

Geriatricians

These are doctors whose training focuses on care of the elderly, and they are particularly experienced to handle the relationship between aging, medication use, and bladder changes.

Nurses

Taking care of OAB and other bladder-control issues is a basic part of nursing practice, as nurses provide care for patients of all age groups and their practices span all types of medical settings. Many advanced nurses, called nurse practitioners, have developed a specialty in the area of OAB and related pelvic conditions. They perform evaluations and provide specific programs for the rehabilitation of pelvic floor muscles and the bladder. They can also prescribe medications and recommend management through the use of catheters, leakage-control products, and devices. Nurse practitioners can practice independently or in collaboration with physicians.

Other Therapists

Other medical providers, such as physical therapists (PT) and occupational therapists (OT), are really physical retrainers. They work with people to help them regain physical function and strength after strokes, heart attacks, accidents, and injuries. Physical therapists may teach Kegel exercises and use biofeedback therapy to strengthen pelvic floor muscles.

Finding Specialized Practices

Over the past decade, specialty practices that concentrate on bladder and pelvic health have sprung up across the United States. Typically, they are headed by primary care physicians, urologists, or urogynecologists and/or nurse practitioners. Providers in these practices perform physical, vaginal, and rectal examinations, pelvic tissue and muscle examination, urinalysis, and more complex tests. Up-to-date treatment plans—behavioral therapy, pelvic-muscle rehabilitation, electrical stimulation, and bladder retraining—are offered in these practices. Providers in these specialty practices are in the forefront of raising public awareness about OAB and related bladder control problems and educating the public about OAB treatments. We have such a practice called the Penn Center for Continence and Pelvic Health at the University of Pennsylvania in Philadelphia. It is unique because of its emphasis on the problem of bladder and pelvic disorders, including OAB. The Center includes a urologist who specializes in women with complex bladder disorders. When seeking help for your OAB, you may want to find a practice similar to ours in order to get the most up-to-date medical care. The National Association for Continence (NAFC) has a list of Continence Experts. Call 1-800-BLADDER (the NAFC hot line) to get the name of a provider in your geographical area. (See appendix B for other resources that may be of help.)

Obtaining a Medical History

Treatment of OAB depends on the severity of your medical condition. The cornerstone of the diagnosis will be the history of your symptoms and other medical problems. The physical examination and test results must be correlated to your history in assessing your urinary problem. Based on the description of the problem and the pattern of the OAB, the characteristics—onset, frequency, and severity—will be noted and evaluated. Your medical provider should thoroughly and carefully question you about your symptoms and urinary habits. Bring your Bladder Diary so they can review your day-to-day patterns with you. You should be able to describe all of the symptoms in detail. The following are components of the history:

- Duration and characteristics of your OAB

- The most bothersome symptoms

- Time of day when the urgency, frequency, and incontinence occurs

- Frequency, timing, and amount of urine leakage

- Presence of factors that precipitate incontinence—laughing, coughing, exercise, effects of surgery, recent illness, or medications

- Whether you experience a sense of incomplete emptying

- Any straining to urinate

- Daily fluid intake

- Bowel habits, such as type and frequency of bowel movements

- Changes in sexual habits (for instance, avoidance of sexual intimacy because of fear of OAB)

- Number and type of absorbent pads used for protection

- Previous treatment and its effect on your OAB. Especially important is any previous pelvic or back surgeries

- Your expectations and goals of recommended treatment. Persons with OAB may want to be totally dry (no urine leakage) or have normal urinating patterns. However, others may feel treatment is successful if they can return to their daily routines, even though they still have some degree of OAB. Talk with your medical provider about what you want out of treatment so that both of you are striving for the same results.

As part of your medical history, you'll be asked questions about any pelvic-floor relaxation or weakness. Symptoms of pelvic floor relaxation include a bearing-down sensation, bilateral (both sides) groin pain, low back pain, difficulty and discomfort during sexual intercourse, any protrusion from the vagina, or difficulty with having a bowel movement.

All related urinary symptoms and habits are important and will be part of your medical history. Lower urinary tract symptoms (LUTS) can be classified as "obstructive" or "irritative." Obstructive symptoms often require referral to a urology specialist, whereas irritative symptoms can often be controlled by routine medical treatments (like drug and behavioral therapy). Obstructive symptoms include:

- ♦ Hesitancy or difficulty starting the urine stream, which causes an increase in the length of time between when you start to urinate by the relaxing of your urethral sphincter and when the urine stream actually begins

- ♦ Bearing down (pushing out) or straining to urinate

- ♦ Dribbling which is being able to urinate only in drops or in an unsteady or decreased flow

- ♦ Intermittency, or stopping and starting of the urinary stream due to the inability to complete urination and empty the bladder on one single bladder contraction

- ♦ The sensation of incomplete bladder emptying

- ♦ Irritative symptoms include:

- ♦ Nocturia, which is awakening at least twice during the night to urinate

- ♦ Frequency, or voiding too often, usually more than eight times in a twenty-four hour period

- ♦ Urgency, or the a sudden and intense desire to urinate

- ♦ Nocturnal enuresis, which is the involuntary loss of urine during sleep. This term is most often applied to bedwetting in children.

- ♦ Dysuria, or pain, discomfort, or a burning or smarting sensation during urinating

Your medical provider will ask you about specifics in your medical history that have a direct effect on the causes of OAB. Significant components in your history which may relate to your OAB include:

- ♦ The number of pregnancies and births, weight of children, episiotomy, use of forceps or vacuum, vaginal or Caesarean delivery

- ♦ Radiation therapy to the pelvic area

- ♦ Prostate surgery, prostate enlargement

- ♦ Reoccurring urinary tract infection

- ♦ Urethral dilations

◆ Previous bladder treatment and the results for incontinence and other bladder conditions

◆ Previous pelvic or vaginal surgery; women who undergo hysterectomy are 40 percent more likely to suffer from OAB-related incontinence as they grow older

◆ Current medications including over-the-counter medications, laxatives, sleeping pills, vitamins, and prescribed medicines can all affect the bladder and need to be noted

At any age, bladder function depends on adequate mobility, memory, manual dexterity, and a healthy lower urinary tract. Part of the examination should include actually watching your ability to use toilet facilities. The ability to reach and use the toilet appropriately is a basic skill for normal bladder function. The time needed to reach the toilet, to undress, and to position oneself for correct urination should be observed. If you are physically disabled, transfer skills (how well you can get on and off the toilet) are important. Your medical provider may ask you to demonstrate how you manage this.

An assessment of memory should be a part of the evaluation of the older person. If memory loss is present the person may fail to grasp the significance of signals of urinary urgency or the social consequences of incontinence. Special kinds of mental examinations can be performed to determine any significant memory loss. During a mental assessment, the medical provider will attempt to determine if you comprehend questions and can interpret sensations.

The Importance of a Physical Examination

To determine the existence and extent of an OAB problem, the abdomen, pelvis, rectum, and nervous system need to be carefully examined. During the more general assessment, your medical provider will check for lower extremity edema, which is swelling in your legs, ankles, and feet. Edema contributes to the increased flow of fluids through the blood while you're lying down or during sleep. During these periods, fluid is reabsorbed into the vascular system, causing increased urine production from the kidneys to the bladder. Many times this increased amount of urine will contribute to the OAB symptoms of nighttime urgency, frequency or nocturia, and nocturnal enuresis. Your medical provider should look for any neurologic abnormalities by checking your reflexes. Neurologic conditions like multiple sclerosis, stroke, or spinal cord compression can interrupt or weaken the nerve pathways to the lower urinary tract, causing the bladder to lose urine or not empty completely.

As you know, manual dexterity is necessary to successfully use toilet facilities. Your medical provider may ask you to pull your clothes up and down and fasten and unfasten buttons, belts, zippers, snaps and hooks. If a person has difficulty with disrobing, there may not be enough time to prevent OAB incontinence episodes. Simple movements like reaching for the toilet and wiping may be difficult for older adults or disabled persons. Also, your medical provider may want to observe you put on an incontinence product that you need or use.

An examination of your abdomen (stomach) is performed to detect the presence of bowel sounds, masses, bladder fullness, or tenderness above the pubic area. Bowel sounds may be absent if you have a bowel problem like constipation. Bladder fullness (called *distension*) may suggest that the bladder is not emptying completely.

In women, a pelvic examination will be conducted where the woman lies in a comfortable position with her legs raised and separated, knees bent. In women, a complete pelvic examination allows a medical provider to determine the presence of atrophic changes (wasting away of muscles and tissue), pelvic organ prolapse (dropping or falling of pelvic organs—uterus, bladder, rectum), perineal (area between the thighs) skin rashes or redness, and any changes in the vagina, uterus, or bladder. Women who have changes in the tissue inside and outside of the vagina complain of burning when urinating, itching, and urinary frequency. These symptoms can lead to OAB. Women with large fibroids in their uterus can have OAB symptoms. In women who have been through menopause, loss of color, dryness, and tenderness in the area of the vagina and urethra are indications of a deficiency or lack of the hormone estrogen. Women with pelvic organ prolapse may complain of urinary urgency and frequency and describe a bulging feeling in their vagina. If you have a prolapse, your medical provider may want to also examine you standing. In this position, the prolapse may become more pronounced. The different types of pelvic organ prolapse are:

♦ *Cystocele:* the tissue between the bladder and the vagina has lost its tone and allows the bladder to protrude (drop) down into the vagina. It's really a form of hernia, and like a hernia, the cystocele can become worse with time

♦ *Uterine prolapse:* the uterus and cervix bulge into the vagina. This often occurs with a cystocele.

♦ *Urethrocele:* the descent of the lower part of the urethra out the urinary opening (urinary meatus).

♦ *Rectocele:* is the bulging of the posterior wall (back part) of the vagina against the rectum, which lies behind it.

Most women have some degree of shift of the organs in the pelvic area, which may not relate in any way to OAB. Childbirth, heavy lifting, chronic straining during bowel movements, and loss of estrogen contribute to pelvic prolapse. A *pessary,* a non-surgical treatment, can be used for pelvic support. This device is inserted in the vagina and rests against the cervix, similar to the contraceptive diaphragm.

It's important to determine the strength of the pelvic floor muscle during the pelvic exam. Weak pelvic muscles may contribute to or cause urinary urgency. Your medical provider will ask you to tighten your muscles during the vaginal examination by squeezing or pulling in and upward with her vaginal muscles in fast contractions called "flicks." When asked to contract the pelvic muscle, many women will either use muscles other than the pelvic muscle or will bear down or push as they do during a bowel movement.

In men and women, a rectal exam is performed to check for painful hemorrhoids, stool impaction (hard stool in the rectum), rectal sphincter tone, and sensation. If a man or woman has a weak rectal tone or decreased sensation, this can cause fecal incontinence.

Women are examined lying on their backs with knees bent. In men, the rectal examination is performed with the man lying on his left side with his knee bent. In men, a genital examination is performed to evaluate skin condition and detect abnormalities of the foreskin, glans (head) of the penis, and perineal skin. This type of examination is important to determine if there is any skin breakdown, swelling, or enlargement of the penis. In men, the rectal examination should also include an assessment of the size, consistency, and contour of the prostate. A large prostate may prevent the bladder from completely emptying, leading to OAB. If an abnormal or enlarged prostate is discovered, the man should be seen by an urologist. It's also important to check the pelvic muscle tone in men.

Medical Test and Terms

An evaluation of OAB should include a urinalysis to check primarily for infection and blood in the urine, and the observation of urine leakage or weighing of incontinence pads, where the medical professional determines the amount of leakage by observing you in leakage-provoking actions and weighing your soiled incontinence pads (see next section). An additional test called a *post void residual* (PVR) may be necessary to see if you are able to completely empty your bladder. There are more complex tests called urodynamics that may be completed in certain instances. *Urodynamics* are a set of tests to measure the function of the lower urinary tract, (the bladder and urethra), by determining bladder capacity, the ability of the bladder to fill and empty, and determining the position, length and mobility of the urethra. Many specialists perform urodynamic tests using sophisticated computerized equipment. However, the goal of all testing is to reproduce the symptoms that you report and to correlate these symptoms with testing.

Urinalysis is the only test that should be part of your first visit to a medical provider. It measures the amount of blood, sugar, protein, and bacteria in your urine. Specimens for urine testing are collected by having you urinate into a container. Blood in the urine occurs when the bladder wall and muscle become irritated, usually by an infection, stones, or a tumor. A person with hematuria (blood in the urine) must undergo further testing to rule out the possibility of bladder cancer. Elevated sugar in the urine usually indicates diabetes. Bacteria in your urine may be a sign of infection, and you may have symptoms of frequency, urgency, dysuria, lower abdominal or pelvic pain, nocturia, pyuria (pus in the urine), incontinence, and low back pain. Any infection should be treated before beginning therapy. If an infection is suspected from the urinalysis, a urine culture will be sent for laboratory analysis. If the culture is positive, showing the actual cause of bacteria in your urine, you will be placed on antibiotics for five to ten days.

When Further Tests Are Necessary

A urinalysis is usually the only test that should be done if you have a simple OAB problem. People requiring further evaluation and tests include those who have failed to respond to treatment, have hematuria (blood in the urine) without infection, have chronic conditions such as a stroke or multiple sclerosis, are experiencing recurrent urinary tract infections, report difficulty with bladder emptying, or who are found to have severe pelvic organ prolapse or an enlarged prostate during an examination. There are many specialized diagnostic tests available. You will probably not need to have these tests, but we want to provide you with a brief description of them.

Pad Test

Weighing and counting pads, often referred to as a "pad test," may be recommended by your medical provider if you have incontinence. You will be asked to collect your urine-saturated pads in a plastic bag for a twenty-four-hour period and bring them, with one dry pad, to the provider's office. The saturated pads are weighed, and the weight of the dry pad times the number of saturated pads you used that day is subtracted from the total weight of the saturated pads. This provides the quantity of urine leakage you experienced for that day.

Provocative Stress Test

Directly observing any urine leakage (called a provocative stress test) is done in a medical provider's office. You must have a full or nearly full bladder before this test is done, so you may be asked to drink several glasses of water to fill your bladder, or your bladder may be filled with sterile water through a catheter. You will be asked to cough vigorously three times and bend and bounce on your heels while the medical provider looks for urine leakage visually or through the use of a small pad. If leakage occurs at the time of your cough or is delayed by a few seconds, this suggests stress urinary incontinence. If the leakage does not occur immediately, you may have OAB.

PVR

PVR or a *post-void residual urine volume* is a measurement of the amount of urine left in your bladder after you urinate. The bladder never totally empties. There is always a small amount of urine left in your bladder. Have you ever become engrossed in a book or magazine story while on the commode? Usually you stopped in the bathroom to urinate and find some peace and quiet from household demands. You urinate and get caught up in reading and before you know it, twenty minutes has passed, your foot has fallen asleep, and you find yourself urinating a few more drops or ounces. That's normal! Normal range of residual urine is up to one to two ounces, but in older people it may be higher. A PVR measurement should be performed to ascertain if the bladder is completely emptying. *Urinary retention* is when a person is unable to empty their bladder completely or at all. There are two main causes of urinary retention: decreased bladder contractions or urethral obstruction. In addition, constipation that causes a large amount of stool in the lower colon or rectum can cause compression on the urethra, thus preventing the bladder from emptying. An enlarged prostate or a cystocele (dropped bladder) that compresses the urethra can also lead to obstruction. A PVR volume should be obtained within five to ten minutes after you urinate, and anything over five ounces left in the bladder can be considered abnormal. People who have abnormal PVRs and who have repeated bladder infections may need to see a specialist. Measuring the PVR volume may involve repeated measurements to be sure of accuracy. One method of PVR volume measurement is catheterization where a catheter (a thin, soft, flexible tube) is inserted through the urethra into the bladder. A safer method is using a bladder ultrasound or bladder scan.

CMG

A *CMG* test determines the ability of the bladder to fill, store, and evacuate urine. It also evaluates the presence of urge sensation. If you have severe urgency with a relatively low bladder volume (less than ten ounces) and/or urine leakage occurs, it may suggest that you have OAB. During the test, you lie on your back on an examination table and a catheter is inserted. Once the catheter is in place, water is instilled through the catheter at a set pace, while the machine records bladder pressure. Normally, bladder pressure rises slightly as instillation begins, then remains at a low, constant level while the bladder fills. The bladder pressure will rise very slightly as the bladder reaches capacity, at which time you will get an urge to urinate. You are asked to report your first sensation of feeling or sense of bladder fullness, which is called the initial urge. A person usually has the first sensation of filling at three to seven ounces of water. Then you will be asked to tell when you feel a strong urge, usually felt at seven to thirteen ounces of water. Very strong feelings of urinary urgency occur at ten to eighteen ounces. When filling and recording are finished, the bladder is drained and the catheter is removed.

Uroflow

One of the simplest, noninvasive tests is the *uroflow* (uroflowmetry) in which urine flow rate is directly observed as you urinate. The curve of the urine flow when urinating is considered helpful in identifying abnormal urination patterns, especially in men who may have an enlarged prostate constricting the urethra. Ideally you should have a full bladder when this test is performed. During the test you will urinate in a funneled container while the curve of urination is electronically recorded by a timer under the commode. The uroflow test measures how long it takes you to start to urinate, the strength and smoothness of your urine stream, the total time it takes you to urinate, and how you stop urinating. If there is a delay in initiation of urination and prolonged urination, you may have a problem with urethral obstruction.

UPP

Urethral pressure profilometry (UPP) measures function of the urethra. This is determined by inserting a catheter into the urethra and measuring or recording the resting and dynamics pressures in the urethra while the catheter is slowly withdrawn (pulled out). A UPP may be more helpful for women.

Cystoscopy

Cystoscopy is a procedure that allows the medical provider to look into your urethra and bladder. A thin telescope as well as a catheter are inserted into the urethra and bladder and your bladder is filled with sterile water. Then, the urethra will be inspected for any strictures (blockage or scar tissue), and the bladder is examined for any stones, infection, or other abnormalities. The doctor can identify bladder lesions and foreign bodies, as well as urethral diverticula (pouches or sac openings), fistula (abscesses), or scars.

The previous chapters have provided information on the problem of OAB, how your bladder works, related problems, completing a diary, and components of a history and examination. There isn't just one solution to resolving your OAB, and there are a number of possible treatments currently available. Choosing the right one may be complicated because each individual's response to a treatment is different. Treatment regimens have advantages and disadvantages depending on a person's age, medical condition and length of condition, previous treatment, and personal wishes. The attitude of the public, doctors, and nurses toward OAB can also affect treatment. The next four chapters discuss the current treatments for OAB. Read and learn about these treatments so when you talk with your medical provider you will have the tools to make a treatment decision that's right for you.

Chapter 8

Your Diet and OAB

When you seek a solution for your OAB, your medical provider will generally recommend a combination of two successful treatments: drug therapy and behavioral training programs. Combining these two treatments will increase the chance of improving OAB symptoms. These treatments are simple and generally have minimal side effects. Usual drug therapy for OAB consists of the use of anticholinergic/antimuscarinic medications. Behavioral training, including self-care practices, bladder retraining, and pelvic-floor exercises are usually the first method recommended to help OAB. Behavioral training without drug therapy may be a valuable alternative for older adults who are at greater risk for developing side effects and complications from drug therapy.

Behavioral training assumes that you have learned maladaptive patterns or behaviors (bad habits) of urinating that may contribute to your condition and its severity. The goal of a behavioral training program is to teach you to relearn or regain bladder control.

The best way to learn new behavior, or to re-learn old behavior, is by identifying the desired behavior and gradually outlining the steps to be taken to achieve the desired behavior. This shaping or outlining is achieved through goal setting and positive reinforcement or reward. During a behavioral treatment program you will be asked to keep a Bladder Diary for at least 3 days as discussed in chapter 6 to monitor your urinating patterns and specified behavior. A critical part of any behavioral program is feedback from your medical provider on your progress and the tips they provide on how to achieve success. There are several different behavioral treatments, including self-care practices such as modifying your diet by maintaining adequate fluid intake and avoiding foods that contain bladder irritants. Other treatments include bladder retraining and pelvic muscle exercises or Kegels. The first step in your treatment process is to identify everyday practices that may be adversely affecting your bladder. Let's begin by discussing your diet.

Diet and Your Bladder

Most medical providers, doctors, and nurses dealing with OAB start treatment with the least invasive, nonsurgical techniques—self-care practices, bladder training, drug therapy, and Kegel exercises. Only if these measures don't work do more complicated, invasive treatments come into play.

The goal of any treatment for OAB is to reduce or eliminate symptoms and to improve your quality of life so you can start doing the things you used to do. Self-care practices such as adequate fluid management and avoiding foods and beverages in your diet that contain bladder irritants are the first steps to reducing your urgency and frequency and in some cases urine leakage.

Adequate Fluid Intake

Like the millions of Americans who have bladder-control problems, people with OAB often think that reducing the amount of liquids they drink will lead to less urine and thus less urination. Decreasing one's daily fluid intake is more common than you might think. Surveys of urination habits of working women have shown that these women drink less while working to decrease their urination frequency. One needs to understand that adequate fluid intake is necessary to eliminate bladder irritants and actually help prevent OAB. Consider Rosemary's story.

Rosemary, a recently retired sixty-four-year old lady, came to our office eight months ago complaining of "dark, smelly urine." Her urinalysis and culture indicated that she had a UTI and she was treated with antibiotics. She returned two months later with the same complaints, and again, her urine culture was positive for infection. We prescribed more antibiotics and also gave her a Three-Day Bladder Diary to complete and bring in with her when she returned for her follow-up visit. During a review of her Diary, we noted that Rosemary was only drinking three to four glasses of water or juice a day. When we suggested that this was a very small amount of fluid, Rosemary mentioned that she was a babysitter for her three-year-old grandson. She felt she had to limit her drinking so that she could reduce her trips to the bathroom, because she can't leave him alone when she urinates.

Rosemary may be correct in thinking that drinking less liquid will result in less urine in her bladder, but this isn't a good thing to do. While drinking less does decrease the amount of urine your kidneys produce, it also causes more concentrated urine. This smaller amount of concentrated urine can irritate the lining of your bladder. Highly concentrated (dark yellow, strong smelling) urine may actually cause you to go to the bathroom more frequently. It can also encourage bacteria to grow in your bladder, which can lead to a UTI. A bladder infection can cause urgency, frequency, and incontinence—all OAB symptoms. Do not limit your fluids to control your OAB unless you're on fluid restriction specifically prescribed by your doctor.

An adequate intake of liquids is especially important for older adults who typically have a decrease in their total body weight and are at increased risk for dehydration. People who live in nursing homes tend to be chronically dehydrated, since most require assistance from staff to eat and drink. Limiting your fluid intake will not eliminate your OAB, and will likely make you constipated, which may result in a more serious problem or illness.

The recommended daily fluid intake for older adults is fifty ounces, but many feel that a more appropriate intake is sixty to sixty-four ounces. Older persons should drink at least fifty to sixty ounces a day. If you are dieting, you may drink extra fluids in the range of 133 ounces a day.

Drinking large quantities of liquids can also cause OAB! Women and men may drink large quantities of water as part of a diet or exercise program. That is why completing a Bladder Diary and reviewing it with you medical provider is so important, as you may have habits that are adversely affecting your bladder.

The times of day you drink can also be a factor in your OAB. Drinking a large volume of fluid at one time, such as at mealtime, forces the bladder to cope with more liquid than it's used to in a brief period of time. This filling leads to an overwhelming sensation of urgency. Spread your intake throughout the day, avoiding high volumes at any one time. The timing of fluid may be particularly important if you have a problem with nocturia. Nighttime incontinence, called nocturnal enuresis, can be a particular problem for your family especially if a family member must get up to assist with toileting. Efforts should be made to maximize the sleep period. To help you minimize your nocturia, follow these simple measures:

◆ Decrease your intake of fluids in the evening by drinking the majority of fluids before 6 P.M., shifting your fluid intake from the evening to the morning and afternoon.

◆ Eliminate all alcohol and foods and beverages containing caffeine from your evening meal.

◆ Take a one-to-two-hour afternoon nap with your legs elevated to the level of your heart using a stool or pillows. This will allow fluid that has pooled in your tissues to flow back through your blood to the kidneys. You will increase urine output during the day, thus decreasing the need to void at night.

Eliminating Bladder Irritants

Yes, there is a relationship between your bladder and what you eat. Certain commonly ingested foods and beverages contain ingredients that can irritate your bladder muscle, causing OAB. We want to tell you about a recent visit to our office from someone who had first hand knowledge of this relationship.

Maria is a nurse in our hospital. She works in the intensive-care unit on the night shift, twelve hours from 7 P.M. to 7 A.M. In order to stay alert and be ready for any crisis, she needs her coffee. Maria loves coffee, the stronger the better. She also drinks several cans of Mountain Dew during her shift. The only problem is that when Maria gets home in the morning and tries to goes to sleep, she has to get up several times to urinate. Maria wonders if the coffee is causing her frequency.

We suggested that Maria stop or cut back on the amount of coffee and soda. You may be wondering why. Well, if you have problems with urgency, frequency, and incontinence, we recommend that you decrease or eliminate certain foods and beverages from your diet. These include products that contain caffeine, alcohol, and sweetener substitutes that contain aspartame (like Equal or diet products).

Caffeinated products have three compounds that affect the bladder—caffeine, theophylline, and theobromine, all of which are part of a group of chemicals called *methylxanthines*. Methylxanthines act as a diuretic—they increase urine production. Caffeine can also cause a significant increase in bladder pressure, leading to urinary urgency and frequency. Theophylline is usually found in tea, and theobromine is in cocoa or milk chocolate. Those seniors who drink lots of coffee and tea are more likely to complain of urinary frequency with subsequent urge incontinence.

Over 80 percent of the population consumes caffeine in the form of coffee, tea, or soft drinks on a daily basis. In the U.S., caffeine consumption is estimated to average approximately 200 mg daily, which is equivalent to the amount in two eight-ounce cups of brewed coffee. Caffeine occurs naturally in coffee beans, tea leaves, and cocoa beans, and the concentration of caffeine in these products is dependent on the preparation method. Nutritional supplements, puddings and desserts that contain cocoa (like pudding or cakes) are favorite foods and daily staples in institutionalized settings like nursing homes. Additionally, the U.S. Federal Drug Administration (FDA) has listed more than a thousand drugs that can be bought over-the-counter in pharmacies and drug stores that contain caffeine. Caffeine content is usually listed on the product label. Table 1 is a list of food products and drugs that contain caffeine.

Medical research has shown that OAB symptoms decrease if you reduce your caffeine intake or switch to caffeine-free food products (Tomlinson 1999). If you want to see if caffeine has an effect on your bladder, eliminate it from your diet for one week and see if your urgency and frequency decrease. Keep a Bladder Diary, and check your results! It may be necessary to gradually replace caffeinated beverages or foods with non-caffeinated ones. Since caffeine affects the nerves and can reduce blood flow to the brain, a sudden withdrawal from caffeine can cause headaches, nervousness, nausea, and muscular tension, so we recommend that you gradually decrease your caffeine intake.

Some specific foods and beverages (carbonated drinks, tomato based products, highly spiced foods, citrus-based juices and fruits) are thought to sometimes contribute to OAB. Alcohol should also be avoided as it acts as a diuretic and can irritate the bladder, causing urgency and frequency. Their effect on the bladder is not always understood but you may want to eliminate one or all of the items listed and see if your bladder control improves.

This chapter provided you with some simple but important strategies that are under your control to try to see if you can decrease your OAB. In our practice, we recommend these to all our OAB patients. However, there are some more treatments so read on.

Table 1: COUNTING CAFFEINE

Hot Beverage	Milligrams per Eight-Ounce Cup
Coffee, Brewed	100–164
Coffee, Instant	50–75
Coffee, Decaffeinated	2–4
Tea, 1-Minute Brew	20–34
Tea, 5-Minute Brew	39–50
Hot Chocolate	2–15

Cold Drinks	Milligrams per 12 Ounces
Iced Tea	67–76
Coca-Cola	46
Diet Coke	46
Tab	49
Pepsi-Cola	43
Diet Pepsi	36
Jolt Cola	71
Dr Pepper	40
Mountain Dew	54

Chocolate Baking	Milligrams per Ounce
Milk Chocolate	1–15
Sweet, Dark Chocolate	20
Baking Chocolate	25–35

Over-the-Counter Medications	Milligrams per Tablet
Anacin	32
Excedrin	65
Midol	32
Darvon	32
No-Doz	100
Vivarin	200

Other	
Chocolate	25 mg per candy bar

Chapter 9

Retraining Your OAB

As we reviewed in chapter 8, behavioral modification, like changing your diet, is considered the most appropriate initial treatment for OAB. Modifying your diet and maintaining appropriate liquid ingestion and bowel regularity are the first steps in overcoming your OAB. The next step is learning how to "retrain" your bladder and how to identify and exercise your pelvic-floor muscles. Bladder training, sometimes referred to as bladder re-education or retraining, teaches you to how to restore your normal pattern of urination. To do this, you follow mandatory scheduled urinating times and gradually adopt longer time intervals between urination. Bladder retraining can help you correct habits of frequent urinating, increase your bladder capacity, and teach you to take control of strong urinary urgency. The ultimate goal of this treatment is to return you to normal bladder function. Contraction of your pelvic-floor muscle can decrease urinary frequency and urgency and prevent incontinence.

As part of bladder retraining and pelvic-floor muscle exercise treatment, it's important that you understand your brain's control over your lower urinary tract, especially your bladder and pelvic-floor muscle. To help you achieve a more normal urinating pattern of every four or five hours, you will learn how to control your urgency by using "urge inhibition" techniques. These techniques include relaxation methods and distraction techniques that involve concentration on an idea or image. Another technique that you can use to control urgency is pelvic-floor muscle contractions. Gaining control over your bladder and pelvic-floor muscles will lessen the likelihood of urine leakage.

This treatment may sound simple, but it requires your active involvement for it to be successful. Research on bladder retraining and pelvic-muscle exercises has shown its success in women with OAB symptoms (Burgio 2001, 2002). In addition, the research shows that with retraining, your bladder begins to hold more urine and thus you will not feel as though you need to go to the bathroom as often.

Understanding Urgency

If you have OAB, the "urge" probably controls you! You can regain that control by performing a behavioral treatment called bladder training. Here's Amelia's story:

> *Amelia is sixty-one and works as an executive secretary for a partner in a large and busy law firm in Philadelphia. Amelia has noticed that for the last five years she has been visiting the ladies room more frequently. This is a problem because the restroom is on the third floor and Amelia works on the fourth floor. Amelia usually takes the stairs because the elevator is slow and Amelia has started to feel a real immediate and intense urge to get to the bathroom. But it is hard for Amelia to "rush" down those stairs. In addition, her bladder urges are happening more frequently, causing Amelia to be away from her desk more often. It seems that the receptionist who covers Amelia's phone when she's away is getting annoyed. Amelia is frustrated because she doesn't seem to have a problem when she's at home or when she's asleep. What can Amelia do?*

First, in order to begin the retraining process, you must understand your symptoms, so let's review them. OAB symptoms include urinary urgency, frequency, and in most cases urge incontinence. Frequency is urinating often, usually eight times or more during day and nighttime hours. Most times the actual urine volume is small amounts. Frequency can worsen if you get into the habit of urinating "just in case," which means that the bladder never fills completely and holds only a small amount of urine. It is better to wait until the bladder is full then empty the bladder. Frequent urinating actually decreases the amount the bladder is comfortable holding.

People with OAB go to the bathroom more frequently because of urinary urgency. Urgency is a feeling or sensation that you need to urinate. It may occur suddenly and may be uncomfortable. The urgency may be so intense that you may feel you need to go immediately or risk having a urinary "accident" on the way. In chapter 2, you learned that the urge is a nerve message from your brain telling you to urinate. Your bladder may be full and ready to empty, or it may not be full, but may be contracting and trying to empty anyway.

Often we hear our patients say "When I gotta go, I gotta go." They feel, as you may feel, that there's no choice. But this isn't really true. When you first feel the urge, you do not have to immediately go to the bathroom. The urge feeling is only telling you that urinating is necessary, not that it has to occur immediately. If you have OAB, you have probably lost the ability to wait, to make your urgency subside or stop. However, you can retrain your bladder to hold and wait.

The Urge Wave

The normal urge feeling comes in waves and follows a pattern. (See Figure 6). The urge starts, grows, peaks, and then subsides until it stops. If you're like most people with OAB, you'll rush to the bathroom as the urge grows and when it peaks you may have an urge incontinence episode if you don't make it. You may feel that the faster you run, the better. But once you start allowing the urge to control you, you will find yourself rushing to the bathroom the moment the urge comes on. You may even find yourself losing small amounts of urine as you get there. The key to controlling the urinary urge is *not* to respond by rushing to the bathroom. Rushing causes movement, which jiggles your bladder, which, in turn, increases the urge feeling.

In addition to rushing, there are other things that can increase your urge to urinate. Seeing a sign for a restroom, hearing running water, going from a warm to cold room, and even seeing the bathroom itself can trigger your desire to urinate. From childhood you have associated the bathroom with urinating, so if you already have an urge to urinate, approaching the bathroom is likely to increase your urge and make urine leakage more likely to occur. If you are experiencing incontinence as part of your OAB, the worst time for you to go to the bathroom is when you have a strong urge, as the movement of rushing or hurrying to the bathroom can cause a

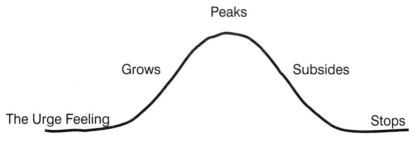

Figure 6: The Urge Wave

bladder contraction leading to urine leakage. It's better for you to practice strategies discussed below for controlling the urge, making the urge lessen in intensity or having it go away.

Identifying a Urinating Schedule

Bladder retraining requires developing a relationship between you and your medical provider. A complete bladder retraining program can take six to eight weeks or more before you achieve success. Your urinating schedule is followed during the day; no schedule is expected to be followed during sleeping hours, and your provider must take into account your lifestyle and preferences when helping you create your schedule. For instance, since Amelia's problem seems to occur more during work hours, her bladder retraining program will target her behavior during those hours. Once a urinating schedule has been identified, she should make every effort to stick to the schedule exactly as prescribed and not to urinate off schedule, even if she experiences urgency. What should you do if you get the urge to urinate and it's not part of your schedule? You practice strategies for controlling urgency. You learn how to relax!

To help you understand your urinating patterns, you need to keep a Bladder Diary in your journal for at least three days. Based on these records, your medical provider will prescribe a urinating schedule, usually suggesting a trip to the bathroom every thirty to sixty minutes. You will be asked to make every effort to stick to this schedule during the daytime. Ultimately the goal is to gradually increase the time between bathroom visits. Every week you will increase the time between bathroom visits by fifteen minutes. So, for example, after one week you would increase the time between urinating to one hour and fifteen minutes. Then at your third week, you would increase to one hour and thirty minutes. Each week you are encouraged to increase the intervals between urinating by fifteen minutes until you get to an interval of every four to five hours. How can you do this? By controlling your urge.

Bladder Battles—Controlling the Urge

Learning to relax can counter your strong urge feeling and allow you to wait longer before using the bathroom. You can then stop the bad habit of frequent urinating, improve your ability to stop urine leakage, and cut down on urinary urgency. You may think that the only way to relieve your feeling of urgency is to urinate and empty your bladder, but this is not so. Urges come and go without emptying your bladder. Remember they are simply messages and *not* commands. You need to think of your urge as a warning only.

Deep Breathing

To help you control the urge to urinate, concentrate on another body sensation. We suggest you try a slow, deep breathing exercise, which is a distraction method to interrupt the bladder urgency message from the Bladder Control Center in your brain. By practicing deep breathing, you will find that the urgency lessens or even disappears. First, when the urge comes on, try to practice these deep-breathing steps:

1. When the urge comes on, stop what you're doing and sit or lie down comfortably.

2. Relax by taking five deep breaths, inhaling deeply and slowly through your nose.

3. Concentrate on the air moving in and out of your lungs, your chest and belly moving in and out.

4. Place your hand on your stomach to feel it expand while you inhale.

5. Purse your lips and slowly and steadily exhale until your lungs have completely deflated.

Repeat this exercise ten times each time you get the urge to urinate. You will be more successful if you try this first in a low stress situation such as when you are at home with the bathroom nearby.

Distraction

A second technique is to use mental-distraction strategies such as concentrating on an activity or a mind game, for example counting backwards from 100 by sevens, listing the birthdays of brothers, sisters, and other close family members, or reciting the words of a favorite song or nursery rhyme.

Quick Flicks

A third technique is to tighten your pelvic muscle *quickly* and *hard* several times in a row. These types of muscle contractions are sometimes referred to as "quick flicks." Usually, bladder training is combined with pelvic-floor muscle contractions to enhance the success of behavioral treatments. You will learn more about how to tighten your pelvic-floor muscle later in this chapter. Note how long you are able to keep the urge away using this method.

Back on Schedule

Once the urge has lessened in intensity or is gone, you should try not to urinate for at least ten to fifteen minutes. If you get a strong urge and it is not your scheduled time, practice your urge controlling techniques and make every effort to wait until your assigned time. If you're concerned about having an incontinent episode, do go and urinate, but after that go back to your scheduled times. If this occurs often, discuss it with your provider to see if your schedule needs adjustments. You may need to have less time between urinating.

Always try to decrease strong urge sensations before urinating. Once the urge has lessened or disappeared, then walk, unhurriedly—*do not run*—to the bathroom to urinate. In order to reduce the chances of awakening during the night to urinate, empty your bladder immediately before going to sleep. Also, remember to cut down on caffeine and beverages and foods containing alcohol.

Try not to be discouraged by setbacks. Sometimes during periods of increased stress, such as attending an important social event where a restroom is inaccessible, you may experience a setback and revert back to old habits. Do not despair! Just pick up your schedule once the stress has been resolved.

How do you know if you're successful? Keep a Bladder Diary throughout the retraining process to monitor if you are urinating less often during the day and if you're having less OAB. Your medical provider will want you to bring these records when you return for visits so they can be reviewed and successes can be identified.

Tips to Follow for Successful Bladder Training

Let's review those things that can help make sure your bladder retraining is successful.

- ◆ Upon awakening in the morning, the first thing you should do is go to the bathroom and empty your bladder.

♦ Use deep breathing to distract and relax your bladder when you have the urge to urinate more frequently than your scheduled time. For example, if you get the urge to urinate whenever you start to unlock your front door, often referred to as "key-in-the-lock syndrome," stop, relax, and take five slow, deep breaths until the urge lessens or passes. Then unlock the door and walk slowly to the bathroom.

♦ Do not urinate before you get the urge.

♦ Walk slowly to the bathroom. Rushing, running, or any fast movement may increase the urgency and precipitate some urine leakage.

♦ If you find you're waking up to urinate more than once during the night (nocturia), do not drink liquids after 6 p.m.

♦ Always believe you will be successful.

Let's read what Amelia did.

Amelia decided to talk with her gynecologist about her urgency problem. Amelia had an examination, and her urine was checked for possible infection. Amelia's gynecologist felt that her bladder and pelvis seemed normal and referred her to a practice that specialized in providing behavioral treatments. The specialists taught Amelia bladder training techniques that included deep breathing once the urge came on. Her new doctors stressed to Amelia that breaking the pattern of immediately responding to an urge and running to the third floor was the goal. Amelia was also taught pelvic-floor muscle contractions to use at the time of urgency. At first, they instructed Amelia to keep to a schedule only in the morning. Once she became successful, she extended her scheduled urinating times to include the afternoon. Amelia was not always successful, and it took two months, but these specialists had such an attitude of positive expectation that Amelia began to believe that success was possible—and she found that her hopes come true.

Amelia was able to control her urgency and decrease her frequency by practicing bladder retraining. She also was able to use pelvic-floor muscle contractions to control her urgency. Now let's discuss your pelvic-floor muscle and how you can use it to control your OAB.

Learning About Your Pelvic-Floor Muscle

As we mentioned, pelvic-floor muscle exercises, often referred to as Kegel exercises, can decrease your symptoms of OAB, particularly urinary urgency and urge incontinence. The aims of this treatment are to:

♦ Prevent a detrusor muscle contraction by voluntary contracting the pelvic-floor muscles when you have the urge to urinate

♦ Counter the fall of pressure in the urethra that occurs with an involuntary bladder contraction

Unfortunately for women, the normal cycles of human life often bring on an overactive bladder. As we've discussed, childbirth, the aging process, and loss of estrogen at menopause cause weakening of pelvic-floor muscles, damage to the bladder neck, and shifting of the uterus. Women with OAB need to be aware of the functions of their pelvic muscles. In chapter 2 we discussed the role of the pelvic floor as a strong, flexible muscular structure, often described as functioning like a hammock. The pelvic-floor muscle has striated muscle fibers that are under voluntary control and can be exercised. The pelvic floor surrounds, suspends, and anchors the pelvic organs, helping them remain in place. These muscles contract and expand during urinating and bowel movements. They also distend during and contract after childbirth. In men, the pelvic muscle surrounds the prostate and external urinary sphincter. Normal bladder function in both men and women is difficult to maintain without the strength and support of the pelvic-floor muscle. Pelvic-floor muscle exercises involve training your pelvic muscles, the goal being to isolate a pelvic-floor muscle, called the levator ani which is often referred to as the pubococcygeus (PC) muscle, (see Figures 8 and 9). By actively exercising pelvic-floor muscles, OAB symptoms, especially urgency and incontinence, improve.

The urethra is closed by the urethral sphincter and the surrounding pelvic-floor muscles, mainly the PC muscle. This muscle consists of two types of muscle fibers, categorized as "slow twitch" and "fast twitch," which are controlled by the pudendal nerve. *Fast twitch* muscle fibers produce strong, rapid muscle contractions when exercised, which are needed to produce powerful contractions during a cough or sneeze. Fast twitch muscles will fatigue if exercised for long periods of time. *Slow twitch* fibers generate a less intense, sustained contraction and are useful to build muscle strength.

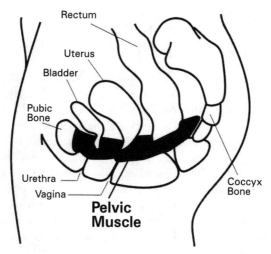

Figure 8: Female Pelvis

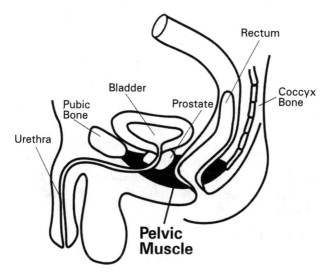

Figure 9: Male Pelvis

Contracting the PC muscle lengthens and compresses the urethra and maintains the angle between the bladder and urethra in its proper position. Strong pelvic-floor muscles decrease the problem of frequent urination and the feeling of urgency. Repeating pelvic exercises on a regular basis increases the force and duration of bladder contractions.

Pelvic-Floor Muscle or "Kegel" Exercises

Kegel exercises or pelvic-floor muscle exercises were introduced around 1948 by Dr. Arnold H. Kegel, a California gynecologist. The exercises were originally designed for women with stress urinary incontinence. Once women performed these exercises, they saw such dramatic improvements in incontinence that Dr. Kegel regularly began to teach the exercises and, as the saying goes, the rest is history. Since Dr. Kegel first described his exercises, they have become the first option for people with mild to moderate stress urinary incontinence and have also been shown to be helpful to people with urgency and urge urinary incontinence. Improvement in symptoms has been shown to occur in 60 to 80 percent of cases. Doing Kegel exercises also has other benefits. The PC muscle is the muscle that contracts during orgasm, so exercising this muscle may make women more sexually responsive. Men also find that building their pelvic floor muscle strength leads to firmer erections and more powerful orgasms.

Kegels are sometimes labeled as ineffective. They've gotten this bad rap due to two simple reasons. Often they have not been properly taught and learned and the need for the continued, regular use of Kegel exercises is not reinforced. Many women are taught to do Kegels, but are unsure if they're doing them correctly. Anyone who tries to do these exercises must take them seriously and have the commitment to practice them. Studies have shown men and women, young and old, have benefited from the exercises. But it is necessary to be motivated and determined to work for the significant benefits possible. Kegel exercises:

- Are not hard to do
- Take time and effort to learn
- Must be done regularly, several times a day
- Can be done anywhere and at any time

Dr. Kegel described four phrases that are seen during a pelvic-floor muscle exercise program:

- Awareness of the function and coordination of the PC muscle. For seniors and people whose pelvic muscles are severely relaxed, this may take several weeks.
- Gains in muscle control.

♦ Improvement of the symptoms indicates that the muscles are strengthening. At this point, some people feel that their incontinence is so improved that regular exercising is no longer needed. This is generally not true.

♦ Firmness, thickening, and broadening of the muscles.

These are the steps you want to achieve by doing Kegel exercises.

Beginning a Personal Kegel Exercise Program

Cathy has been experiencing urine leakage for several years. At first it was just a nuisance, only occurring once or twice a week and only in drops. But, in the last couple of years it has started occurring more frequently especially every time she laughs, has a bad cough, or runs on the treadmill. Several years ago, her gynecologist told Cathy about some exercises, and she has decided to try them now. The only trouble is that Cathy's not sure she's doing them correctly. At this point she isn't sure what to do or if she should do anything about her problem.

Cathy should find a medical provider who can help her identify her PC muscle and implement an individual pelvic-floor muscle exercise program. During an examination, she will be helped to identify her PC muscle by "squeezing" or tightening the muscle around the provider's finger. This enables the provider to determine the exact strength of the pelvic-floor muscles. Pictures of the pelvic-floor muscles and nerves will give you a clear idea of placement of the muscles within the pelvic region so that you know which muscles to control. In addition, detailed oral and written instructions should be included in this process.

There are several ways to find your pelvic-floor muscle, and we've described each one separately. You should be alone in a quiet place where you can concentrate and experiment. After you figure out each technique, take several minutes to try it. If the first technique doesn't work for you, go on to the next. It doesn't matter which technique you use to find your pelvic-floor muscles, because the muscles tend to work as a group. So squeezing one of the pelvic floor muscles indicates that the others are working, too. When women contract their pelvic-floor muscle when sitting, they'll feel a slight pulling in the rectum and vagina. When men do so, they will feel a pulling in of the anus and movement of the penis. Every person is unique, and different techniques work for different people.

♦ *Technique 1:* Everyone at one time or another has been in a crowded room and felt as if he or she were going to pass gas or "wind." Imagine that this is happening to you. Most of us will try to squeeze the muscles of our anus to prevent the passing of gas. The muscles being squeezed are the pelvic-floor muscles. If you feel a "pulling" sensation at the anus, you're using the right muscles. In most of our patients, we have found this to be the most successful technique.

♦ *Technique 2:* If you are a woman, lie down and insert a finger into your vagina. Try to squeeze around your finger with your vaginal muscles. You should be able to feel the sensation in your vagina, and you may also be able to feel the pressure on your finger. If you can, you're using the right muscles. If you cannot detect any movement with one finger, try two fingers.

♦ *Technique 3:* For heterosexual, sexually active women, try to contract your muscle around your partner's penis during intercourse. If you are contracting the correct muscle, your partner should feel the contraction pressure on his penis.

♦ *Technique 4:* For men, stand in front of a mirror and watch your penis. Try to make your penis move up and down without moving the rest of your body. If you can, you're using the right muscles.

♦ *Technique 5:* Insert the tip of a finger into your anus and try to squeeze your finger as if you are holding back a bowel movement. You should be able to feel the sensation in your anus as well as the pressure on your finger. If you can, you are using the right muscles.

You may not find your pelvic-floor muscles immediately. Many people have to take their time with this. Remember, you're searching for muscles that you may not have been aware of before, and your muscles may be weak. So for now your goal is only to locate your pelvic-floor muscles.

Depending on your needs and abilities, your medical provider will schedule office visits to begin supervised pelvic muscle rehabilitation sessions. Initially, frequent sessions are needed so that the provider is certain that you've identified, isolated and are using the correct muscles. At first, it may be difficult to isolate and flex the correct muscles, but the more exercises you do, the easier it will become.

Avoid Exercising the Wrong Muscles

One of the most common mistakes often made is exercising the wrong muscle. When trying to find a new muscle, especially a weak one, most people tighten other muscles too. Some people clench their fists or teeth, hold their breath, or make a face. None of these actions really help. It is very tempting to use other muscles, especially stronger ones, to support smaller, weaker muscles such as the pelvic-floor muscles. However, using other muscles interferes with learning how to use the right ones. It is best just to relax your body as much as possible and concentrate on your pelvic-floor muscles.

The most commonly used "wrong" muscles are the muscles of the abdomen (stomach or belly). Most people who are learning to control their pelvic-floor muscles tense their belly muscles at the same time. This happens so often that the muscles may seem to be connected. They are not. It's very important to separate the muscle groups and to keep your abdominal muscles relaxed while you squeeze your pelvic-floor muscles. When tightened, abdominal muscles raise the pressure in your bladder and actually make it more likely that you will leak urine. Abdominal muscles tend to push urine out of the bladder instead of holding it in.

To avoid using your stomach muscles, rest your hand lightly on your belly as you are squeezing your pelvic-floor muscles. Do you feel your belly tightening? If you do, relax and try again. Be sure that you do not feel any movement in your stomach.

Are you holding your breath? If you are, you're probably using your chest muscles. First, relax completely and notice how you are breathing for a few moments. Then squeeze your pelvic-floor muscles while you continue to breathe normally. This will help to assure that you are not using your chest muscles, because chest muscles are usually relaxed when you breath.

The other set of wrong muscles are the muscles of the buttocks (bottom). To test whether you're also tightening your buttock muscles by mistake, squeeze your pelvic-floor muscles while sitting in front of a mirror. If you see that your body is moving up and down slightly, you are also using your buttock muscles.

Another set of muscles commonly used are the thigh muscles. If you see your upper legs moving, which will cause your entire body to lift, you are contracting the wrong muscles. When done properly, no one should be able to tell that you are squeezing your pelvic floor muscles—except for you.

If you cannot find any of your pelvic-floor muscles, consult your medical provider for assistance with this step. Once you have found the muscles, even if they are weak, read on.

Once you have the ability to contract the pelvic-floor muscle, you can work with a daily Kegel exercise program in the privacy of your own home. The beauty of the exercise is that it can be done silently and discreetly, while watching television or sitting in front of a computer—any time at all.

Strengthening your Pelvic Muscles

Now that you have located your pelvic-floor muscles and you are able to squeeze them without using any other muscles, you are ready to begin your daily exercise program.

The reason for daily exercise is twofold. First, exercise increases the strength of your pelvic-floor muscles so that they will be strong enough to prevent urine leakage. Second, through repeated practice you gain control over these muscles. Then you can use them quickly to prevent urine loss or to decrease the urge feeling. These exercises are the mainstay of your program.

Learning pelvic-floor muscle exercises can be difficult at first and may require more concentration than you expect. This is true for most new skills. Do you remember learning to read? With a multitude of details to keep in mind, it's hard to imagine reading as automatically as most of us now do. Well, learning to exercise pelvic-floor muscles is also a skill. But with persistence and continued practice, these exercises will become second nature. Soon you'll find yourself doing them automatically.

If at any time you find yourself getting the wrong muscles involved, *stop!* Rest for a moment and start again, using just your pelvic-floor muscles. If you are tired and unable to stop using the wrong muscles, stop and rest. Go back to the exercises later in the day.

Each exercise consists of squeezing and then relaxing your pelvic-floor muscles. Squeeze the muscles for three seconds, and then relax the muscles for three seconds. The easiest way to do this is to squeeze and count slowly, "1 . . . 2 . . . 3." Then relax and again count slowly, "1 . . . 2 . . . 3." A squeeze and relax is considered one exercise. Holding the muscles to a slow count of three is important for increasing muscle strength. Remember, squeeze and count slowly, "1 . . . 2 . . . 3," then relax and again count slowly, "1 . . . 2 . . . 3." Do another exercise. Make sure you hold the squeeze for the full three seconds.

It is common for most people to not take the time to relax between squeezes. You must allow the muscles to relax so that your muscles can rest before squeezing again. Take time to relax to the same count (1 ... 2 ... 3) as you squeeze (1 ... 2 ... 3).

Doing Your Exercise Program

We recommend that you complete at least two exercise sessions a day. Generally, do one set in the morning when you get up and one at night. Do sixty pelvic-floor muscle exercises every day, divided into two sessions of thirty exercises each. Remember, each squeeze and relaxation counts as one exercise. Do the exercises in each of these positions every day: ten exercises lying, ten sitting, and ten standing. The exact time of day is not crucial. What is important is that you develop the habit of doing the exercises every day. You can make this happen by planning your exercise schedule in advance. Choose two times of the day when you can be sure you will always have the time to exercise and you will remember to do the exercises.

It is essential for you to feel comfortable using your pelvic-floor muscles in all positions. The sensation that you will feel while squeezing is different when you are standing compared to when you're sitting or lying down. More important, you may need to prevent leakage in any of the three positions, so you must have control over your pelvic-floor muscles in all positions.

It is felt that one of the best positions for doing Kegels is standing and leaning on a counter top. Many people find that the standing position is the most difficult. Part of the problem is that you are less likely to feel the contraction of your muscles while you are standing. You may think that the muscles are not working properly when, in fact, they are working just fine. Keep trying.

In the beginning, you will need to set aside time to concentrate while you do the exercises. This should be a quiet time, when you're alone and won't be disturbed. Each time should be associated with a cue that will remind you to practice. For example, you may want to exercise just before you get up in the morning and before you fall asleep at night. Any activity that you perform regularly on a daily basis can be used as a cue.

In our office, we provide patients with a Bladder Exercise tape, which leads them through an exercise session of muscle contractions and relaxation. We ask patients to listen to the tape and follow its instructions twice a day. It's always good to have a step-by-step reminder, so we supply them to our patients for use at home. If you like, you can make one of these tapes yourself, recording three sets of ten exercises. Or you can ask a friend or family member with a pleasing voice to record it for you.

Remember to do thirty exercises at each session. Doing the exercises in sets of thirty assures that the muscles are getting strengthened. Doing fewer exercises at each session, even if they total sixty for the day, may not exercise the muscles adequately. If you tire before you reach thirty, rest briefly and then finish the session.

Are you worried that it will take too much time? If you are squeezing and relaxing to a slow count of three, a session of thirty exercises will take you about three minutes.

When you are counting "1 . . . 2 . . . 3" at the same time that you're counting exercises, you may lose track of how many exercises you've done. If you find this happening to you, you can set a timer for the total time you expect to be exercising. Since you will be squeezing and relaxing to a slow count of three, you should set the timer for three minutes.

If you'd like to do more than sixty exercises each day, feel free to do so. But before you do more, make sure you are squeezing the correct muscle. Pelvic-floor muscle exercises cannot hurt you—they can only help. In fact, most people who have overcome OAB with this method report that they also exercise whenever they think about it throughout the day (in addition to their scheduled sixty exercises). When it occurs to them, they simply squeeze their muscles a few times to keep in practice. Try to do three or four exercises whenever you walk to the bathroom, stand up from a chair, are driving in your car on your way to work, when you stop at a red light, are standing in line at the grocery store, or whenever the telephone rings. Squeezing your pelvic-floor muscles whenever you think of them helps to make their use easier and more automatic in your daily life. No one will know that you are using them except you.

Remember, your pelvic-floor muscles will be weak in the beginning. Like any other muscle, they need some time to gain strength. Many people give up after only several days of practice, because they see no change. Pelvic-floor muscles need more time. You will probably see improvement after the first two weeks, but the muscles may not reach their full potential for at least six months.

Soon, after two weeks of exercise, you will find yourself able to hold the squeeze comfortably to a count of three for the full thirty exercises.

Cathy spoke with her gynecologist about her feeling that she was not contracting the correct muscle. He taught her during her pelvic examination how to identify and tighten her muscle.

Cathy has been doing the exercises for two weeks, squeezing the muscle for a count of three. She feels that her muscle is getting stronger. Her husband doesn't even know she is doing them. Now she's ready to hold the "squeeze" longer.

To develop the muscle strength and bulk, you will need to extend the time you squeeze and relax your muscle from three to ten seconds. The reason for this progression from three to ten seconds is to ensure that your pelvic-floor muscles get stronger and bulkier, allowing them to stay "squeezed" for a longer period of time. You need to gradually increase the time you hold the muscle, so it may take you four to six weeks to get to ten seconds. We recommend that you start to hold for five seconds the third week. Remember to squeeze and count slowly, "1 ... 2 ... 3 ... 4 ... 5" then relax and count, "1 ... 2 ... 3 ... 4 ... 5." You can increase the number of exercises you are doing each day from sixty to ninety. Here is an exercise schedule to follow:

- Lying down squeeze for five seconds and relax for five seconds, fifteen times

- Sitting down squeeze for five seconds and relax for five seconds, fifteen times

- Standing up squeeze for five seconds and relax for five seconds, fifteen times

Each set of fifteen exercises will take about five minutes to complete. So an entire exercise will take you around fifteen minutes. If you do these exercises twice a day, (ninety exercises), it only takes thirty minutes out of your day. At week five, increase your muscle squeezes to ten seconds. Remember to squeeze and count slowly, "1 ... 2 ... 3 ... 4 ... 5 ... 6 ... 7 ... 8 ... 9 ... 10" then relax the muscle and count, "1 ... 2 ... 3 ... 4 ... 5 ... 6 ... 7 ... 8 ... 9 ... 10." Continue with forty-five exercises, twice a day. We do not recommend doing more than a total of ninety exercises a day unless recommended by your medical provider.

Using Your Pelvic Muscle to Control the "Urge"

Many people think that the only way to relieve the uncomfortable feeling of urgency is to empty your bladder, but you will see that this isn't so. Urges can come and go without your emptying the bladder; they are simply messages telling you that eventually you will need to urinate. In someone with OAB, the urges are often false messages that you need to go *now*. Urges are not commands. They should function as an early warning system, getting you ready to find a place to urinate—after you have relaxed and suppressed the urge.

To reduce the urge to urinate, you will use your pelvic-floor muscles. Remember to squeeze your pelvic-floor muscles quickly several times when you get the urge feeling. To do this, tighten/squeeze and relax the pelvic muscle as rapidly as possible. Do not relax fully in between squeezes. Try this now. Squeezing your pelvic-floor muscles in this way sends a message to your bladder to stop contracting. As your bladder stops contracting and starts relaxing, the urge feeling subsides. Then, once the urge to urinate has subsided, you have a safe period when the bladder is calm. This calm period is the best time to go the bathroom.

These Exercises Cannot Harm You

These exercises are not harmful. You should find them easy and relaxing. If you get back pain or stomach pain after you exercise, you are probably trying too hard and using your stomach muscles. If you experience headaches, then you are also tensing your chest muscles and probably holding your breath. We do not recommended that you practice these exercises during urination by starting and stopping the flow of urine. It can be harmful to try to stop your flow of urine while urinating when bladder pressure is high, pushing the urine out of your body.

Pelvic-muscle support usually improves within one month after starting the exercises and six weeks should bring significant changes. However, symptoms improve slowly, so tracking symptom improvement is essential. Keeping a Bladder Diary in your journal is an excellent way to track your and identify the success of the exercises.

Making These Exercises Part of Your Life

Make the exercises part of your daily lifestyle so that exercising becomes a habit, almost like a reflex action. After six weeks of practice, the exercises will require less effort, and you will no longer need to set aside special times to concentrate on them. Tighten the muscle when you walk, before you cough, as you stand up, and on the way to the bathroom. Try to always tighten your muscle when you get a strong urge that you cannot control. Do your exercises when:

♦ Standing at the sink and brushing your teeth

♦ You get up in the morning

♦ You're washing dishes

♦ Putting on your make-up

♦ Sitting in the car at a stoplight

♦ You're having dinner

♦ Reading a book in bed

♦ Watching TV—during each commercial

♦ Going for a walk

♦ Talking on the phone

♦ Having sex

Do your exercises during your daily activities or routines. Once you have learned how to do the exercises, increased you pelvic muscle strength, and improved you OAB symptoms, you don't have to keep a formal count of the number of times you do each exercise—just do it several times in a row. Do them often enough to make them a habit. Remember, the more exercising you do, the:

♦ Stronger your pelvic floor muscles will get

♦ Faster they will get stronger

♦ Easier it will be to maintain muscle strength

Advanced Assessment Techniques

If a person has weak muscle tone, there are various therapies and devices that may aid in performing pelvic-muscle exercises. These can be taught by providers such as doctors, nurses, or therapists who specialize in pelvic-muscle rehabilitation. Dr. Arnold Kegel, the gynecologist who first described pelvic-floor muscle exercises, developed the *perineometer*, a pressure-sensitive (similar to a balloon) device that is inserted into the vagina to help women identify and train their pelvic-floor muscles. By inserting this device into the vagina, the force of Kegel exercise contractions is measured. A woman can then adjust her exercise pattern so that the exercises are performed correctly.

Since Dr. Kegel described the benefits of using a device to assist with these exercises, several tests have been developed to measure pelvic muscle activity. A test called the *electromyogram* (EMG) measures activity through electrodes placed on the skin surface or through sensors inserted into the vagina or rectum. Manometry has now replaced Dr. Kegel's perinometer. *Manometry* (balloon measurement) testing is performed by inserting devices called *pressure sensors* into the vagina or rectum. When contracting your muscles, the sensor or electrodes, identify your pelvic-floor muscle contractions. EMG and manometry are used to test the strength of your muscle contraction.

Biofeedback therapy is all about learning your body's signals. For over thirty years, this therapy has helped people use the processes and functions of their bodies to improve health problems. You probably use biofeedback every day if you step on a bathroom scale to find out your weight. The scale provides the feedback to you about your body's weight. Biofeedback therapy is a dynamic process, really a type of information transfer. We are usually unaware of many of the processes of our bodies—heart rate, blood pressure, and certain types of muscle control, because they seem automatic. We go on our merry way and all of a sudden our blood pressure soars; our heart rates get faster; we're "stressed out" and suffer pounding headaches; we get ulcers trying to cope with daily pressures; we leak urine. Biofeedback to the rescue! It teaches a person to hear and listen to what the body is saying to them. For instance, you can use biofeedback to raise or lower heart rate and blood pressure or reduce stress and headaches by learning relaxation techniques. In other words, you learn to listen to your body and change your habits according to what you learn.

The goal in using biofeedback as a treatment for OAB is to alter the responses of the detrusor and pelvic muscles that control urine loss. Biofeedback can teach you how to control the external sphincter by using a device to measure the action of the pelvic-floor muscles and "feed back" to the person information about how well the muscles are performing. Biofeedback therapy is usually performed in one of the two ways mentioned above, electromyographic (EMG) or manometry. The method you may be offered depends on what equipment your provider has.

A balloon device (the EMG sensor) or electrodes on the skin are used to measure electrical signals from the sphincter and muscles. The information is stored, processed, and "fed" back to you in a variety of ways. Information about the status and condition of pelvic-floor muscles, nerves, and bladder function is immediately accessible and can be interpreted simultaneously by the provider and patient.

Your motivation and active participation play a big part in the success of biofeedback therapy. Biofeedback therapy can be performed when you're lying down, standing up, or sitting in a chair. The position will depend on your provider and your progress. For people with bladder-control problems such as OAB, biofeedback therapy uses computer graphs or lights as a teaching tool to help you identify and learn to control the correct muscles. Biofeedback helps you locate the pelvic muscles by changing the graph or light when you squeeze or tighten the right muscle. Optimal biofeedback therapy includes visualization of both pelvic and abdominal muscle movement, so in addition to using electrodes on the skin or a sensor in the vagina or rectum, skin electrodes may be placed on your lower belly to see if you are contracting muscles other than your pelvic muscle.

Using Weights to Strengthen your Pelvic Muscle

Weights that are put in the vagina can be used by women to strengthen pelvic-floor muscles. They've been most successful in women with stress urinary incontinence and are often used as part of pelvic-muscle exercise programs. The weights are shaped like tampons and come in sets of increasing heaviness. Each weight has a nylon string attached through the end that helps the user remove it. The tapered portion is inserted first. If your medical provider thought weights would be of benefit to you, you would assume a semi-squatting position or stand with one foot on a chair to facilitate insertion of the weight. You would insert the lightest weight into the vagina, in the position of a tampon, then walk around for up to two minutes. If the weight is retained during this time, you would introduce the next heaviest cone, and repeat the procedure until one slips out. Once identified, you'd use that weight, holding it in by contracting the pelvic-floor muscles for up to fifteen minutes, twice a day. When you can successfully hold that weight, you would move up to a heavier one. If you're able to keep the weight in place, you know that you are using your pelvic muscles correctly. Holding the contraction required to keep the weight in the vagina strengthens pelvic floor muscles. It is advisable to wear underwear while using the weights.

Vaginal weights are designed for one-person use, and careful washing and drying between use will ensure the necessary cleanliness. These weights are generally used by women of all ages, but shouldn't be used during menstruation or if the woman has a urinary tract infection. A pelvic-floor exercise program should be performed in addition to the use of weights.

Stimulating Your Pelvic Muscle to Contract

Applying a low-grade electrical current to pelvic-floor muscles stimulates the pelvic muscle to contract. This treatment is called *neuromuscular stimulation* and may be a useful addition to pelvic-floor exercises in the rehabilitation of weakened pelvic muscles. It can be very beneficial for men and women who are unable to contract these muscles on their own because it can teach the correct action. The electrical currents stimulate and contract the same muscles as Kegel exercises. The difference is that voluntary compliance is not required. Stimulation is applied to the body using skin electrodes around the anus or sensors inserted in the vagina or rectum. Stimulation is usually combined with biofeedback. Electrical stimulation heightens the perception of the pelvic-floor muscles and biofeedback will show you the muscle contraction as it is stimulated.

There are no side effects to electrical stimulation of the pelvic floor, but it shouldn't be used if a woman is pregnant or has a heart pacemaker. Electrical stimulation is sometimes performed in the provider's office as part of biofeedback therapy or by the use of a small battery operated unit that the person uses at home. If you have a home unit you will be instructed to use the stimulator one or more times a day for several weeks to several months. Electrical stimulation is usually combined with a pelvic-muscle exercise program.

This chapter provided a very detailed review of how to perform bladder retraining and pelvic-floor muscle exercises. In chapter 8, you learned about how to make sure that your diet and daily liquid intake do not contribute to OAB. These behavioral treatments can improve your OAB symptoms by over 50 percent allowing you to lead an active and productive life. However, to achieve the greatest chance of successfully improving or eliminating your OAB symptoms, combining *both* behavioral and drug treatments is the best option. Chapter 10 will provide you with the newest in drug treatments.

Chapter 10

Drugs That Can Help OAB

It's important that you learn all about your treatment options, so ask your medical provider about them before you decide which is best for you. With all treatments discussed in this book, you should ask about the advantages and disadvantages, the risks and benefits of each. Also, be sure you understand your medical provider's reason for suggesting a specific treatment. But the final decision is yours. Remember:

- No single treatment is right for everyone.

- No single treatment works for everyone.

- Every treatment has advantages and disadvantages.

- Nobody can predict or guarantee how you will respond to any given treatment.

For these reasons, most medical providers usually combine treatments, particularly behavioral and drug therapies. These are the most readily available and frequently offered treatments. Depending on either your symptoms or the result of your evaluation, OAB can be treated in this manner.

Actress Debbie Reynolds spoke about her personal experiences related to bladder health at the *Women's Forum on Lifelong Pelvic and Bladder Health* sponsored by the National Association for Continence. She related her problems with OAB and her positive experience with one of the available drugs.

Sue also has an OAB problem, and her story may have some similarities to yours:

Sue is a healthy sixty-year-old lady who is slightly overweight. She is usually up six to seven times during the night to urinate and, during the day, urinates at least every hour. Sue had a terrible thing happen to her when she and her husband were at the symphony. In the middle of the first movement, Sue had a very intense need to urinate. She excused herself and had to crawl pass six persons in her row to get out to the bathroom. She urinated, went back into the concert and within fifteen minutes had another strong intense urge. She again excused herself and crawled past six persons to get out of her row and go to the bathroom. When she returned, she had to go again within thirty minutes! This time, her husband became very angry, people in her row made it even more difficult for Sue to get out. Sue was so embarrassed. This time when she got to the bathroom she had wet herself. She decided to leave for home without her husband.

Sue has OAB symptoms. If OAB is caused by contractions of the bladder muscle (detrusor overactivity), drugs called anticholinergics or antimuscarinics, which reduce bladder muscle contractions, are prescribed.

Drugs used to treat OAB affect the nerve and muscle function of the detrusor muscle, cause the detrusor muscle to relax and thus reduce the frequency and intensity of contractions of the bladder. They can also increase bladder capacity.

These drugs work by blocking the attachment of a neurotransmitter called acetylcholine to specific sites on the bladder muscle (called receptors). The attachment of neurotransmitters to the receptors sets in motion a sequence of changes that results in muscle contractions. Blocking this combination prevents the contraction. Because of these two actions, these drugs are called antimuscarinic or anticholinergic agents (they are the same thing).

The receptors to which the acetylcholine attaches are found, however, not only in the bladder but in other organs as well. The effects in those other organs may occur to a lesser degree but cause the side effects (which are unwanted and undesirable) of the drug. These common side effects are seen in the following organs:

♦ *Salivary glands*—dry mouth

♦ *Bowel*—constipation

♦ *Eyes*—blurred vision, dry eyes

♦ *Heart*—fast heart rate

♦ *Brain*—confusion, memory problems

The goal of all companies making such drugs is to develop a medicine that is truly bladder selective, having few or no significant effects outside of the bladder. These drugs have been tested in adults and have been shown to:

♦ Reduce urine leakage, both frequency and amount

♦ Decrease the feeling of urgency.

♦ Decrease the numbers of times you have to go to the bathroom.

Six to seven out of ten persons with OAB who take drug therapy see an improvement in their symptoms. If drug therapy is combined with the behavioral treatments described in Chapters 8 and 9, persons can see even greater improvement (Burgio 2000).

Drugs for OAB are classified as either immediate-release (IR) which means it works within hours or extended release (provide 24-hour effectiveness) drugs where relief from OAB symptoms can be seen both day and during the night.

Drugs Most Often Prescribed for OAB

Newer medications that target the bladder specifically cause fewer side effects and safety concerns and have greatly improved the management of OAB. At this time, the most commonly prescribed drugs used to treat OAB are tolterodine and oxybutynin (both come as pills and oxybutynin comes as a skin patch as well). There are several drugs that are in development or are being considered by the FDA (Food and Drug Administration) for approval, and we will also mention those.

Tolterodine

The first antimuscarinic/antocholinergic drug to be developed specifically for OAB is tolterodine (brand name Detrol). This drug is found to more specifically affect the cholinergic receptors in the bladder that cause contractions or overactvity. It is found to be more selective for bladder receptors over salivary gland, which means that it has less of the side effect of dry mouth than other currently available oral drugs. Tolterodine is available in both immediate (IR) and extended release (ER) doses. The extended release, called Detrol LA (long acting), is the one most often prescribed. The IR dose is 1 or 2 mg (milligrams) taken once or twice a day, and the ER comes in doses of 2 or 4 mg taken once a day.

It is recommended that you take the long-acting form of the drug at the same time each day. The extended release (ER) formulation of tolterodine (Detrol LA), at a dose of 4 mg every day, provides significant improvements in the symptoms of OAB and is felt to be more effective than the immediate release form, with a lower chance of the dry mouth side effect (Abrams, 1998, Chancellor, 2000).

Tolterodine appears to have fewer of the problems seen with the other oral antimuscarinic drugs currently available for the treatment of OAB.

Oxybutynin

The oldest, commonly used anticholinergic/antimuscarnic drug for OAB is generic (a non-brand or trade drug) immediate release oxybutynin, which has been around for more than twenty yeas. It was originally found effective for urge urinary incontinence in patients with nervous-system disease.It blocks bladder contractions or overactivity by relaxing the bladder muscle. Although it is effective, generic oxybutynin is associated with side effects that are often severe enough to cause persons to discontinue its use. Of particular concern is bothersome dry mouth, which occurs in 61 to 78 percent of patients receiving generic oxybutynin. (Yarker, 1995)

The recommended dosage of generic oxybutynin is 2.5 mg to 5 mg tablets taken three or four times a day, but doses of 2.5 mg tablets taken twice a day are commonly prescribed in older adults. Side effects may develop in persons taking generic oxybutynin and include dry mouth, blurred vision, dry eyes, constipation, and increased eye pressure in persons with glaucoma, heart irregularities, and delirium.

To minimize the side effects and to improve the effectiveness of oxybutynin, different types and routes of drug delivery have been developed. They include an extended-release tablet, which makes possible the slow and steady release of the drug, and a transdermal (skin) patch. Ditropan (oxybutynin) XL is the brand name of the extended-release oxybutynin. XL refers to the extended release of this drug, which is taken once a day and makes possible the slow and steady release of oxybutynin over a twenty-four hour period (Gupta, 1999). This formulation of the drug works well because there is a difference in the site in the bowel where Ditropan XL is broken-down and this results in less production by the gut (gastrointestinal tract) and liver of the compound (or metabolite) primarily responsible for the side effects of the drug (Wein 2001, Anderson 1999). Ditropan XL is available in 5, 10 or 15 mg tablets. Usually a medical provider will prescribe 5 mg, and increase the dose to 10 mg, then perhaps higher depending on the effect the dose has on a person's OAB symptoms and the side effects that occur.

The extended release (ER) formation of the drug is preferred by many doctors, as it minimizes the highs and lows of drug concentration so that you can have twenty-four-hour relief from your OAB symptoms and not experience as many side effects. The extended-release formulation is associated with a significantly less dry mouth compared with the immediate-release (IR) formulation. However, it is important to note that the newer ER formulations of both OAB drugs (Detrol LA and Ditropan XL) control drug fluctuations in your blood, reducing peak drug concentrations and thus lowering the risk of cholinergic side effects (Diokno, 2003).

The extended release medication of oxybutynin should be swallowed whole, as it is contained in a nonabsorbable shell. So don't be concerned if you notice something in your stool that looks like a tablet.

You can take these drugs with or without food. You should not crush, break, divide or chew the extended-release medication. If you have problems with nocturia, taking a dose of the immediate-release preparation an hour or two before going to bed may be helpful.

The third type of oxybutynin is a transdermal system (skin patch) called Oxytrol. Skin patches are becoming more common as an approach to delivering drugs. We now have patches to treat menopause, provide birth control, control high blood pressure, decrease chest pain and deliver nicotine to persons who are trying to stop smoking. The Oxytrol patch delivers the active drug ingredient (oxybutynin 3.9 mg each day) through the skin and into the bloodstream. As this drug delivery bypasses the gut (gastrointestinal tract —stomach and bowel) and liver, side effects are thought to be less (Davila 2001, Dmochowski 2002).

A new patch of Oxytrol must be placed two times a week. To help people remember, patients are instructed to change the patch on the same two days each week.

The most common side effects of any skin patch are skin reactions where the patch is put on—itching and redness (Murphy 2000). Any skin reaction from the Oxytrol patch would be minimized if you rotate the site of patch application. Any redness should disappear within several hours after the removing the patch. If uncomfortable irritation or excessive itchiness continues, tell your medical provider. You can use baby oil to remove any adhesive material that remains on the skin after the patch is removed. Other side effects of Oxytrol could include dry mouth, constipation, abnormal vision, and headache.

The patch should be put on a clean, dry, and smooth (fold-free) area of skin on the abdomen, hip, or buttock. The patch is placed on a different area of the skin each time. The person should avoid the waistline area, since tight clothing may rub against the patch. Areas of the skin that have redness or rashes or are being treated with oils, lotions, or powers that could keep the patch from sticking well should be avoided.

So what did Sue do?

> *Sue started to make excuses for not wanting to attend the symphony. She and her husband had season tickets, so he ended up going alone. When Sue realized she was also refusing invitations to friends' parties she made an appointment with her primary care doctor. Sue told her doctor she was desperate, so he ordered an extended release anticholingeric drug, asked her to complete a Bladder Diary for 3 days and return for a follow-up visit in six weeks. He wanted to talk with her about other treatments.*

Don't expect these drugs to work immediately. Usually you will see an effect in the first one to two weeks but it may take up to eight to twelve weeks to reach the maximum benefit (Wein 2001, Wein and Rovner 2002). But each person's response can be different. So stick with the medication prescribed. Also, remember to work on the behavioral treatments at the same time. Here is a review of what they are:

- ♦ Monitor your diet and cut down on foods and liquids that seem to irritate your bladder.

- ♦ Maintain an adequate liquid intake but don't drink large quantities.

- ♦ Keeps your bowel movements regular.

- ♦ Practice bladder retraining techniques.

- ♦ Use your pelvic floor muscle to decrease urgency and incontinence

Common Side Effects

As mentioned, the problem with the current OAB drugs, as with most drugs, is that they all have side effects. The side effects are usually minor, don't last long and can be managed using simple measures. Don't stop the medication if you think you may have a side effect, but do tell your medical provider, because it's often possible to reduce or eliminate the side effect by changing the dose of the drug. Or your medical provider may be able to treat the side effect or recommend simple ways that you can relieve or cope with it. Be patient, as this may take time.

The most common side effect of the antimuscarinic drugs is seen in the salivary gland, causing dry mouth. Dry mouth can lead to excessive drinking and subsequent worsening of OAB symptoms. Severe cases of dry mouth can lead to tooth decay. But, despite this side effect, most people don't stop the drug because of this side effect. Tolterodine is felt to have less dry mouth side effects than oral oxybutynin.

Another common side effect, constipation, is because of the effect on the muscarinic receptors in the bowel, which decreases the transit time of the bowel. Less commonly seen side effects include blurred vision, dry eyes, running nose, and drowsiness.

Anticholinergics may cause sleepiness or blurred vision, so be careful when driving or operating machinery. In addition, sleepiness may be increased by drinking alcohol.

These drugs are *tertiary amines*, which mean that they are thought to be able to cross into the brain and could cause some problems with memory. This side effect is not very common in most adults but it is felt that these drugs should be monitored closely in older people because of a potential increased effect on memory and related cognitive function in this age group.

Inform your medical provider if you are taking any other medications before one of these drugs are prescribed. That includes any drugs that you are buying without prescription (over-the-counter medications). Some of them may cause problems when taken with antimuscarinic or anticholinergic drugs. These include cough or cold medicines, which can affect urination.

Taking two drugs, which are metabolized by the same body system, can increase the concentration of each drug and magnify their effects. Similarly, taking a drug that inhibits the action of an enzyme responsible for breaking down another drug can significantly increase the level of that drug. Therefore, it is very important to make sure your medical provider knows all the drugs (including drugs taken for other medical problems) you are taking. Drug interaction and the effect of one drug in the breakdown of another can be a real problem.

Be sure to tell your medical provider about *all* your medicine and all your medical conditions, especially if you have any of the following:

- ◆ Uncontrolled glaucoma (increased pressure in the eyes)

- ◆ Liver disease

- ◆ Kidney disease

- ◆ Bladder obstruction (blockage)

- ◆ Gastrointestinal obstruction (blockage in the digestive system)

- ◆ Ulcerative colitis (inflamed bowels)

- ◆ Myasthenia gravis (generalized nerve weakness)

- ◆ Gastric reflux disease or esophagitis (inflamed esophagus, the tube between your mouth and stomach)

Who Should Not Use These Drugs?

Don't use these medications if you have the following medical conditions:

- ◆ *Urinary retention:* bladder does not empty or does not empty completely when you urinate.

- ◆ *Gastric retention:* your stomach empties slowly or incompletely after a meal

- ◆ *Uncontrolled narrow: angle glaucoma* (increased pressure in your eye): tell your medical provider if you have glaucoma or a family history of glaucoma.

- ◆ *Pregnancy:* or breastfeeding, as taking drugs may not be right for you.

Other Drugs Used for OAB

Another type of drug, called imipramine, is sometimes used in some cases of OAB, especially in those persons with nocturia. It is an antidepressant and has a dual action when used to treat OAB. It decreases bladder contractions and increases urethral resistance to urine outflow. Therefore, it may be prescribed for OAB and stress urinary incontinence. The usual starting adult dose is 10 to 25 mg a day, which may be increased to 75 mg over several weeks. As this drug may cause sleepiness (called a sedative effect), it may decrease the OAB symptom of nocturia. It should be noted that imipramine is FDA approved for enuresis (bed wetting) in children but *not* for the indication of OAB. Side effects include postural hypotension (low or drop in blood pressure when changing positions) and heart rhythm disturbances in older people. If this drug is stopped, they should be tapered, which means that the dosage is decreased over several weeks.

Desmopressin (DDAVP) is a synthetic analog of vasopressin, which acts as an antidiuretic (prevents filtering of water by the kidneys). This drug has been used in children who wet the bed at night, as it can decrease the amount of urine produced during the night. This drug has been suggested as a treatment for adults who suffer from the OAB symptom nocturia, as it would promote sleep with fewer trips to the bathroom. However, this drug has risks, which include fluid overload (retention of water), which may be a problem if you suffer from congestive heart failure. It can also result in a decrease of sodium in the blood. So this drug should only be used in certain people and under careful supervision by a medical provider.

New Drugs on the Horizon

As you can see, there are several effective drugs for OAB. But we need more. We need drugs that will:

1. Improve bladder function without interfering with the function of other organ systems (called *uroselectivity* or *bladder selectively*)

2. Decrease bladder overactivity without disturbing normal urination.

There are several new medications in development that are being tested in the U.S. At least three, most likely, will be available by the end of 2004. Thus, there will be more options for OAB management.

Three new orally administered anticholinergics agents have been filed with the Food and Drug Administration (FDA) for approval: darifenacin, solifenacin, and trospium chloride. Each has been demonstrated to improve, in clinical trials thus far, the symptoms of OAB (Wein 2001). Darifenacin and solifenacin may be more selective for the muscarinic receptors in the bladder, thus causing less "side effects" in other receptors in the mouth and bowel. Trospium chloride is a quaternary ammonium (which means it is unlikely to cross into the brain causing memory changes) drug that has been shown to increase the capacity of the bladder to hold urine, decrease bladder overactivity and may have fewer side effects than oxybutynin (Madersbacher, 1995). Each drug will no doubt stake a claim for equal or better efficacy and tolerability than the current market leaders.

The symptoms of OAB are 'felt" because nerve impulses come from the bladder to the control nervous system (spinal cord and brain) and are translated there into these feelings (Kuo, 2003). The impulses can also result in an unwanted bladder contraction and urinary leakage. There is a class of drugs, which can block these impulses going to the nervous system. One such agent, currently under study, is resiniferatoxin (abbreviated RTX). RTX, however, needs to be put directly into the bladder through a catheter. If successful, this will need to be repeated periodically (estimates range from every two to every six months).

Botulinum toxin (Botox) is being used for OAB although is has not been approved by the FDA for this condition. If injected intravenously in large enough doses, it prevents normal muscle contraction by interfering with the release of the neurotransmitter, acetycholine. It is widely used, however, by cosmetic surgeons to smooth out wrinkles. Used this way it is injected directly into the muscle layer under the skin in small amounts. The muscle relaxes and the wrinkles disappear! Botox can also be injected directly into the muscle layer of the bladder. Such use can prevent or decrease unwanted bladder contractions. Botox has been used widely in Europe for treatment of difficult OAB cases and is currently under study at some centers in the U.S. As with RTX type drugs, the treatment effects "wears off" and the injection must be repeated.

The Role of Estrogen for OAB

Topical (applying a drug to a specific body part) use of the hormone estrogen may be used to treat women who have gone through menopause (complete or permanent stopping of menstruation) with vaginal atrophy that is contributing to OAB symptoms of urgency and frequency. *Vaginal atrophy,* called *atrophic vaginitis,* is an inflammation of the vagina that develops when there is a drop in levels of the female hormone estrogen. Estrogen plays a vital role in keeping vaginal tissue healthy so when levels of estrogen decrease, vaginal tissue can become atrophic—thin, dry and smaller in size. It can also cause irritation in the urethra and contribute to OAB symptoms of urgency and frequency. Symptoms of atrophic vaginitis may develop slowly and a woman may not notice any symptoms for five to ten years after menopause begins.

The use of oral estrogen has changed since the Women's Health Initiative (WHI) study reported that long term use of oral estrogen (conjugated equine estrogen 0.625 mg) in women five years after menopause increased the risk of heart disease, stroke, pulmonary emboli (blood clots in the lungs) and breast cancer. However, the estrogen used for atrophic vaginitis is a different drug delivery, local use. Local use of estrogen slowly improves the normal urethral lining and may improve the symptom of urgency. Applying estrogen to the area of the perineum, where the vagina and urethra are located, may also prevent bladder infections. However, any form of estrogen should be used with caution in women who have an increased risk of developing uterine or breast cancer.

Local estrogen can be prescribed as a cream, tablet or ring that is placed in the vagina. Using this type of estrogen drug may have a more rapid effect on the bladder.

Estrogen creams (Estrace, Ogden, Ortho, Premarin) are smoothed onto the skin of the vulva (area outside of the vagina) and inserted into the vagina using an applicator or finger. These creams are supplied in a tube with an applicator, which is filled to a predetermined level and inserted into the vagina. The plunger on the end of the tube is then depressed, depositing the cream in place. Some women will squeeze a "fingertip" of cream on their index finger and insert the cream into their vagina. The usual dose prescribed is 1 to 2 grams inserted nightly for ten to fourteen days then two to three times a week.

The estrogen tablets (Vagifem) are inserted into the vagina using an applicator. The applicator is advanced at least halfway up the vagina and the tablet is released. The usual dose prescribed is one tablet nightly for two weeks then twice a week.

A third form of topical estrogen is a vaginal ring (Femring). The ring is inserted in the vagina and it releases a form of estrogen called estradiol in a consistent manner for three months or ninety days. This soft, flexible ring is placed by a medical provider towards the top of the vagina, near the cervix. It releases the estrogen hormone over ninety days, and then it is replaced.

With all these different forms of topical estrogen, it usually takes two months to see improvement and up to six months to gain the full benefits. None of these forms of local estrogen should interfere with sex.

Reported side effects of estrogen use include endometrial cancer, fluid retention, depression, nausea, vomiting, high blood pressure, gallstones, and cardiovascular effects such as stroke and myocardial infarction (heart attack). But all of these side effects are more common when women are prescribed oral estrogen (pills taken by mouth) than when using local treatments. Estrogen therapy can cause some vaginal bleeding. To prevent any problems from occurring while using local estrogen treatment, you should have a yearly pap smear, mammogram and perform a self breast exam a least once a month.

Choosing the "Right" Drug for OAB

With increasing information about drugs on the internet, through advertising in newspapers, magazines and on TV, individuals like yourself, are becoming more familiar with the names of agents used for treatment of various disorders. People often come to the medical provider's office asking if a particular drug might be "right" for them. How does the medical provider evaluate these drugs and choose his or her favorite for OAB?

Clinical effectiveness is the term we use to combine the notions of *efficacy* (how well does the drug relieve the symptoms of incontinence, urgency, frequency, getting up at night), *tolerability* (the side effects and how bothersome are they) and *persistence* (does the patient want to continue taking the drug). A drug with great clinical effectiveness is obviously the "holy grail" of OAB treatment: highly efficacy, high tolerability, and a willingness on part of the patients to stay on treatment. Each medical provider will choose the drug that seems to them, on the basis of published medical reports and colleagues and patients' opinions, to be likely to have the greatest clinical effectiveness in a given situation.

As you have learned from this chapter, there are many new and exciting drug treatments for OAB. All have limitations, and some are associated with side effects that may reduce their acceptance. However, if combined with other treatments such as behavioral modification, they can significantly improve and even cure OAB.

But what if you are one of those people who have tried these treatments and still have OAB? What else can you do? Read on to discover other treatment options and methods of coping with OAB.

Chapter 11

Other Methods to Treat OAB

There are other treatments and management strategies for OAB that are recommended when drugs and behavioral treatments have been unsuccessful. However, these treatments, which are surgical procedures, are performed only if other treatments have been tried and the person with OAB still has severe symptoms. Management strategies involve the use of products and devices that contain or prevent OAB.

Electrical Stimulation

InterStim, also called *sacral neuromodulation,* is a treatment that uses mild electrical pulses (called electrical stimulation) to stimulate the sacral nerves in your lower back, just above the tailbone. The sacral nerves (specifically S_2, S_3 and S_4) activate or inhibit muscles and organs that contribute to urinary control: the bladder, sphincter, and pelvic-floor muscles.

InterStim is done in two stages, so the success of the treatment on your symptoms can be tested before actually performing the full procedure. The temporary test stimulation is done before implantation of the InterStim. If your symptoms improve by a least 50 percent (decrease in urgency and frequency) or disappear during the test period, InterStim treatment may be appropriate.

To permanently place the InterStim system, an operation is performed. An incision is made over your sacral area (lower back) and a lead (a thin wire with small electrodes at its tip) is placed near the appropriate sacral nerve. The lead and wire are passed under the skin to a small neurostimulator (approximately the size of a stopwatch) that is placed in a "pocket" just under the skin on the upper part of your buttock.

Once in place, you can adjust the stimulator by using the knobs on the unit to slowly increase or decrease the intensity of the stimulation. As with any surgery, problems can occur. For instance, the wire may move as you move. If the wire becomes dislodged or moves away from the nerve, the InterStim will not be effective. Pain can occur at the stimulation/implant site and/or lead site. You can get an infection at the site but you will receive antibiotics at the time of surgery and for ten to fourteen days after the implant. If a woman with the stimulator in place becomes pregnant, the unit should be deactivated and a cesarean delivery may be considered. There is a 33 percent revision rate, which means that additional surgeries may be required because of technical failure of the implanted unit.

Other, simpler types of electrical stimulation have been used with varying success. Stimulation can be applied through electrodes that stimulate nerves in lower leg, thigh, abdominal wall, rectum, and vagina.

Making the bladder larger would seem a logical way to treat OAB that does not respond to simpler treatments. This procedure, called *augmentation cystoplasty* is rarely done for OAB. At present, it requires that the bowel be surgically opened and a piece of the bowel is then placed (or sewn) into the opened bladder to increase the size of the bladder muscle—much like sewing a patch onto a large hole in a piece of fabric. Efforts to grow bladder tissue outside of the body and then use it to make the bladder layer are now underway and will eventually eliminate the need for bowel surgery to accomplish this.

But what if you are one of those people who have tried these treatments and still have OAB or are in treatment but are afraid to go outside your home because you're afraid of having a urinary accident. What else can you do? There are management strategies that involve the use of products and devices, so read on!

Seeking Protection

As we discussed in chapter 3, if you have OAB, you may find yourself staying home or always visiting bathrooms when you travel from your home. You probably fear the embarrassment of possible, unwanted, and uncertain urine leakage or incontinence. This can adversely affect your life. You may find yourself seeking some way to protect yourself from this embarrassment, and there are products and devices that can protect you. This chapter provides you with some information on these products, and appendix A at the end of the book offers contact information for companies that supply these products. Consider Jill's story.

> *Jill urinates ever hour. When she gets an urge, it occurs*
> *suddenly, and she sometimes doesn't make it to the bathroom.*
> *Last week when she was in the supermarket, the urge came*
> *on so suddenly that she wasn't able to make it to the*
> *bathroom. She was glad she was wearing black pants so no*
> *one noticed the wetness. After, that, Jill started using sanitary*
> *pads, but they were often too thin.*

If you have OAB, you may find yourself in Jill's position, using pads especially if you are experiencing accidents. Absorbent pads are called *incontinence products* and are either disposable (throw away after using) or reusable (wash and reuse). They absorb and contain unwanted urine leakage. Incontinence products are generally classified for light, moderate, or severe urine leakage. As there are many commercial brands, it can be difficult to compare them. This chapter will help you choose the correct product for your needs.

Absorbent Products

There are several types of products available including pantiliners, pads, guards, undergarments, protective underwear, adult briefs (sometimes called adult diapers), and underpads. Incontinence products can be a useful way to manage unwanted urine leakage. You may be using these products because of the protection they provide and to prevent yourself from the embarrassment of urine leakage. Others use pads because they have been dismissed rather than treated when seeking help for OAB.

The urine-holding capacity of all absorbent incontinence products varies and is not standardized. The quality and materials used in these products vary widely and there is little research comparing absorbent products. At the present time, product selection is made by the consumer through trial and error and depends on cost and availability. Technological advances may have a significant impact on skin problems. You, the buyer, should understand the product you are purchasing so we recommend you ask your medical provider or pharmacist at the store where you are buying the product to recommend products they know work well.

Most products utilize a super-absorbent polymer that turns the urine into a gel, eliminating the possibility of leakage or odor. New techniques have produced better products that can wick or pull urine away to keep the skin dry and free from irritation. Absorbent incontinence products do assist with management of urine leakage, but if the product is not changed on a regular basis, prolonged pressure on the skin from the wet product traps the moisture in the pores of the skin, contributing to skin breakdown.

Absorbent products "soak up" urine. They protect clothing, furniture, and bedding and allow individuals to maintain their self-esteem and physical comfort. The products are available in all types of absorbency, from thin panty liners, sanitary pads, and adult diapers or briefs to bed and furniture protection products like bed pads. Perineal pads are attached to the underwear or panties with an adhesive strip. Undergarments have elasticized legs with a belt that is attached with buttons or velcro. Protective underwear are absorbent products that slip on like cloth underwear. Briefs or diaper-like products have elasticized legs and have self-adhesive tabs that secure the brief.

For men, there are specially designed pads called "guards" that are held in place inside regular underwear with an adhesive strip. They offer more freedom for men with moderate urine loss.

Incontinence products do contain urine leakage and if you suffer from OAB, they can help you maintain your independence and self-respect. It's estimated that as much as 30 percent of all feminine hygiene pads are purchased for OAB problems, especially by young women who have slight incontinence or stress incontinence.

Disposable incontinence products can be expensive. For a person on a fixed or retirement income, this expense adds a burden to an already limited budget. Cost also forces many people to make their own absorbent pads from tissue paper, towels, washcloths, and so on. Additionally, absorbent products are not covered by Medicare, HMOs, or insurance companies.

Washable, reusable garments have a protective outer layer of plastic that is usually made of vinyl, rubber, or a synthetic moisture-proof material. They can be pulled on, side-snapped, or opened in the front. Many women find cotton underwear to be more comfortable than a full incontinence brief, so they'll use a perineal reusable pad placed in the underwear to collect any urine leakage.

Absorbent products can be helpful during treatment of OAB. However, early dependency on absorbent pads may be a deterrent to seeking treatment as they can give you a false sense of security. Do not allow these products to remove your motivation to seek evaluation and treatment for OAB. Problems can occur from improper use of absorbent products as they can contribute to skin breakdown and infection. To avoid these problems, you should change and discard your pads frequently to limit your exposure to the wet product and eliminate build up of odor. Disposable and washable pads are available in supermarkets and through mail order catalogs. JC Penny and Sears carry their own brands.

Frequently, we are asked by our patients or their family members what is the best product to use for protection. This is difficult to answer because there are many factors to consider when using absorbent products. Considerations include the type and amount of urine leakage, preference, quality and cost of the product, ability for a person to remove the product, and the condition of your skin and its risk for breakdown.

Toilets, Commodes, and Collection Devices

Collection devices "catch" urine and include portable commodes, urinals, and bedpans that you can use as a toilet when the toilet is unavailable or hard to reach. These collection devices can be especially helpful if you have urgency and frequency.

One way to decrease the chance of urine leakage on the way to the bathroom is to make toileting easier. A bedside commode may be the answer. Some have drop arms and adjustable heights to allow for individual needs. There are also wooden rather than metal commodes that can be disguised as an easy chair. There are general areas that need consideration when selecting a commode:

- ◆ Height and weight of the person using the commode

- ◆ Mobility and dexterity, especially if you need to empty and clean the commode

- ◆ Whether you have a medical provider who will write a letter of medical necessity, which will allow insurers to pay for at least one commode per person

Changes in bathroom architecture can also help minimize problems from OAB. Removing the bathroom door and using a curtain or swinging door makes access by a wheelchair possible. Grab bars in the right spot and a toilet-seat adapter makes the toilet safer. At least one grab bar should run parallel to the floor at a height of thirty-three inches from the ground. Also, bathrooms with gravity assisted door closer mechanisms are helpful. If you are redesigning your bathroom to make toileting easier, recommended room dimensions are a minimum of five feet by five feet. Many people cannot open bathroom doors, because they cannot grasp and turn the doorknob. Replacing doorknobs with lever-type devices or disabling the door so that the door opens and closes with a push are good remedies.

Bedside or portable commodes are wonderful, movable toilets that are lifesavers for people who have severe symptoms of OAB. A bedside commode can be placed close to the bed for easy use at night or on the floor of the house that does not have a bathroom. Bedside commodes are lightweight and easy to maneuver, but have solid construction. You can buy or rent one from a medical surgical supply store. It's important that the commode be emptied and cleaned after every use. To minimize the odor and to make cleaning it easier, keep water with a disinfectant in the bucket at all times. To camflouge the commode, you can cover it with an attractive cloth, or place it behind a screen.

A raised toilet seat, attached over an existing seat, significantly eases a person's getting up and down on their own. Seats with grab bars on either side are most often recommended to prevent falling and to aid with rising.

A hand-held urinal is bottle-shaped container that can have two different types of necks. They are useful for people with severe mobility restrictions, particularly when visiting places with inaccessible restrooms, traveling, or those confined to bed. They have handles and can be hung on a bedrail, wheelchair, or walker, or can be laid flat on the bed. There are spill-proof male urinals with large funnel openings to deal with a retracted penis. Often these urinals have a flat bottom so that they can be placed on the bed. The openings in rehab urinals have a flange that extends into the urinal and does not allow backflow even when held almost upside down. Female urinals are a good alternative for women traveling, sitting in wheelchairs or chairs, or who are bed bound. However, female urinals that work are not easy to find.

The following are things to consider when choosing an urinal:

♦ Lightweight plastic urinals are useful for people who have difficulty lifting objects. Steel urinals are very heavy and cumbersome.

♦ Handles should be designed so that a person can hold the urinal. If grip is a problem, rubber around the handle will add extra grip. An extended handle may help if wrist movement is restricted.

♦ Ease of use and cleaning is vital.

♦ A spill-proof design is definitely worth considering.

Keeping Your Skin Healthy

If you have OAB, you may be at risk for developing skin rashes and skin breakdown. Good skin care is very important. If you are concerned about your skin and the damage that can happen from your OAB, or if you are caring for someone with OAB here are some basic steps to follow:

♦ Look at your skin carefully every day, separating any skin folds and looking for rash, irritation, or skin breakdown.

♦ Wash your skin with a mild soap or peri-wash product that will not harm the skin. Always wash your skin after any urine or bowel incontinence episode.

♦ After washing, let your skin dry rather than rubbing with a towel to avoid irritation and skin tears.

♦ Use moisturizers and skin products (barrier ointments or creams) that protect the skin from moisture.

♦ Use incontinence products that keep the urine away from the skin.

♦ If you stay in bed a lot or sit in a chair most of the day, protect your skin from moisture, and do not lie on any areas that are open or have a rash.

♦ If you are caring for someone who does not move, turn them frequently and support them in different positions by using pillows or wedges.

Your skin is usually slightly acidic. The acidic pH is a major factor that helps prevent the invasion of bacteria, particularly yeast and fungus. This is often referred to as the "protective acid mantle" of the skin. The presence of urine or feces on the skin changes its pH, moving it into the alkaline range. Furthermore, the presence of excessive skin surface moisture can contribute to the growth of bacteria that can lead to skin breakdown and infection. When combined with changes in skin pH, the effect can be particularly devastating.

An alkaline pH of the skin also adversely affects the skin, further enhancing the loss of normal skin integrity in the person whose skin is already compromised by exposure to urine and feces. When skin is subject to moisture from urine in combination with fecal matter, further skin trauma is produced when the urea (from the urine) breaks down into ammonia by bacteria in the stool. All of these factors work in concert to weaken the skin. Weakened skin, in turn, is more susceptible to irritation, breakdown, and further skin problems.

Proper use of soaps, skin products, topical antimicrobials (agents that inhibit the growth of germs), gentle pH balanced cleansers, appropriate skin barrier products (like Sween), and effective use of incontinence pads help reduce the presence of urinary and fecal matter and prevent skin breakdown. No-rinse perineal washes and cleansers are convenient, time saving, and effectively remove the urine and/or feces without patient discomfort. These cleansers are also preferred over the popular bar soaps because the cleaning agents and antiseptics used in these formulations are gentler to the skin than those used in bar soaps. Additionally, no-rinse perineal cleansers are pH balanced for the skin, whereas bar soaps are almost always in the alkaline range. Some perineal cleansers are also formulated with topical antimicrobials that may decrease the bacteria on the skin.

Creams, ointments and pastes function as skin barriers. However, the recent advent of clear, solvent-based film-forming skin protectants are an even better alternative then creams, ointments, and pastes. Once applied, they quickly evaporate, leaving a protective film. This clear film allows for air flow but is impervious to external moisture and skin irritants.

Careful and close attention to skin care reduces the occurrence of skin breakdown in persons with incontinence.

Pessaries

As women age, the tissues that support pelvic organs may become overly stretched, causing the pelvic organs to drop and sometimes protrude through the vaginal opening. This condition, introduced in chapter 2, is called "prolapse." Women with prolapse have poor pelvic support, allowing the vagina, uterus, and rectum to descend (drop) below their normal position, often causing OAB symptoms. A woman with a prolapse may complain of urinary urgency and frequency, describe a dripping or bulging feeling in their vagina, or feel as though they are sitting on a tennis ball, they also will report pressure in the pelvic organs. Prolapse is divided into four categories: urethrocele, cystocele, uterine prolapse, and rectocele.

Prolapse is usually diagnosed by a physician who "grades" the prolapse depending on how far the organ has dropped. If you have prolapse, you may find that you have to empty your bladder more often or may have unwanted urine leakage. Childbirth, heavy lifting, chronic straining during bowel movements, and loss of estrogen may contribute to pelvic prolapse.

An operation can correct pelvic prolapse especially a cystocele. However, the most common treatment for prolapse is the use of a device called a "pessary." The word pessary can be found in both Greek and Latin literature. These devices have been reported since the time of Hippocrates who mentioned a pomegranate being placed in the vagina to support a prolapse. It has been found that by placing a pessary into the vagina, OAB symptoms can be relieved.

A *pessary* is a device that looks like a contraceptive diaphragm, but the outside rim is hard. Like a diaphragm, it is put into the vagina and rests against the cervix, lifting or supporting the pelvic organs. More than two hundred different types of pessaries have been invented, but only a few are used today.

Pessaries come in many shapes, but the most commonly prescribed pessary is round. You shouldn't be able to feel the pessary when it's placed inside you. When first inserted, a pessary must be frequently removed, at least during the first month to make sure it is a proper fit, is in the correct position, and isn't causing problems to the tissue in the vagina. This can be done by your medical provider or yourself.

Most complications associated with pessaries are minor. Improper fit is common; it takes time and patience to fit pessaries, particularly in older women. Chronic irritation, ulceration of the vagina, and vaginal fistulas (openings in the walls of the vagina) can occur in women who do not properly care for the pessary or who do not go for regular follow-up visits with a medical provider. If ulceration and abrasion of the vaginal wall occur, the pessary should be changed to a smaller size. Adverse effects include back pain, foul-smelling vaginal discharge, or bleeding. Leukorrhea (white discharge from the vagina) is probably the most common problem associated with pessary use, related to the presence of a foreign body in the vagina. Urinary retention can result if the pessary compresses the urethra into the pubic bone.

A pessary can remain in place for several months and a woman can remove and clean it. Problems are not usual, but can happen if the pessary is misused or forgotten. Women who are pregnant, have an infection in their vagina, or who have had recent vaginal surgery should not use a pessary. The ring pessary can be worn during sex depending on comfort.

External Catheter Systems for Men

Men who have OAB that includes urine leakage may use an external catheter to collect their urine. An external catheter is a soft, flexible sheath that fits over the penis and attaches to a urine-collection bag strapped to the leg. It is also referred to as a condom catheter, penile sheath, or an external male catheter. External catheters are designed to collect urine that leaks from the penis and store it in a bag until it can be conveniently emptied. They are suitable for men suffering with severe urinary urgency and frequency that leads to urine leakage and in circumstances where it would be difficult to make frequent trips to restrooms.

There are several different external condom catheters made of latex rubber, polyvinyl, or silicone. They are attached to the shaft of the penis by one of three different methods:

♦ Hydrocolloid strips have adhesive on both sides and can be applied around the penile circumference. The catheter sheath is rolled up and over the strip and penis and pressed to stick.

♦ Self-adhesive types of external catheters are very popular. These are rolled over the shaft of the penis and pressed to stick. Many of the newest models are made of silicone, which causes less irritation and adverse reactions and are recommended for persons who have an allergy to latex.

♦ Some men use no method of attachment and prefer a nonadhesive condom, using a foam and elastic reusable band fastened with Velcro to secure the catheter. There is no direct skin adhesion.

Since there are several sizes of condom catheters, it's important to buy the right size. All manufacturers that make these catheters have a measuring guide that they will send to you. It's worth trying different systems to find the one that best fits your needs. The catheters are disposable and should not be worn for longer than twenty-four to seventy-two hours. In hot and humid weather, they will need to be changed more often.

Problems include skin rash, maceration (softening of tissue) of the penis, ischemia (diminished blood supply), and penile obstruction. Most problems with these catheters are the result of improper and prolonged use of these devices. Also, men who have neuropathy (decreased feeling in the nerve endings) may not feel the discomfort and pain caused by improper usage. If you are using or plan to use a condom catheter, be certain that you learn how to properly apply it and can recognize the problems that can occur with its use.

Before deciding that this type of catheter is for you, there are a few key questions that you need to answer:

♦ Who will place the condom catheter? Is dexterity a problem?

♦ Does the penis shaft have enough length to support the catheter?

♦ What is the condition of the skin? Does protection, such as a barrier film product, need to be used before using the device?

This chapter provided you with examples of products and devices that can help you manage your OAB.

Chapter 12

The Caregiving Dilemma: Growing Old with OAB

You may be in the position of caring for a family member who has a problem with OAB. Consider the following information, adapted from *Taking Care of Aging Family Members* (Lustbader and Hoogman 1994).

The Demographics of Caregiving

Where do older people live?

- 43 percent have lived in their present home for over 20 years.

- Almost 30 percent live alone (32 percent of women, 22 percent of men).

- 33 percent of men and 50 percent of women over age 65 who are widowed, separated, or divorced live with adult children or other family members.

Who provides care in the home?

- Nearly 80 percent of primary caregivers are women, who provide the majority of hands-on care, like changing incontinence products, catheters etc. Daughters outnumber sons three to one.

- One-third of caregivers are age sixty-five and older.

- Women today can expect to spend eighteen years of their lives helping an aging parent and seventeen years caring for children.

- Over half of caregivers report they are caring for someone with urinary incontinence.

Who lives in nursing homes?

- Less than 5 percent of those sixty-five and older live in nursing homes, but more than 25 percent will be in a nursing home at some point during their later years.

- Over 70 percent of nursing home residents are women.

- Almost 10 percent of older people living in private homes would require nursing-home placement if family support were withdrawn.

- At least 50 percent of nursing-home residents have urinary incontinence and, 48 percent have fecal incontinence.

- If you go into the nursing home continent, you have a 39 percent chance of becoming incontinent by two weeks after admission.

Helping A Family Member with OAB

The elderly population is skyrocketing as baby boomers age. This aging population is already demanding better solutions to the health care problems they face. One of those problems will be OAB.

Mr. P.'s daughter brought him to the family doctor's office because she couldn't deal with his stubbornness over refusal to wear an incontinence product. Mr. P. is ninety-two, suffered a stroke a year ago, and has weakness in his right side. He has urgency and needs to urinate at least every two hours. At night, Mr. P. wakes his daughter three to four times a night so she can help him to urinate. He is so embarrassed that he has stopped visiting his friends at the senior center and no longer goes for lunch. The daughter has put pressure on him to wear a product so he can go out of the house. Recently, Mr. P. was taken to the emergency room because he was dehydrated. He had stopped drinking water and juice so he wouldn't have to go to the bathroom as often. The daughter is frustrated and angry with her father, and she is thinking about placing him in a nursing home.

Mr. P. is not unusual. Men with OAB tend to be more finicky about being away from home. Consider that men who must wear a disposable diaper or disposable undergarment can't easily hide spare diapers in a large purse or bag. Men are embarrassed when they have to change their diapers or pads and deposit soiled diapers in trash cans in front of other men in public restrooms. On the other hand, public ladies rooms have small garbage cans in each stall for feminine hygiene product disposal.

For people living at home or in a nursing home, OAB can be a significant burden as they are dependent on others. They are care-dependent and it is costly. Kenneth Langa and colleagues (2002) noted that caregiving by family and friends of older people who have the OAB symptoms of incontinence can be a substantial cost. Assessment and treatment of OAB in people, who are frail, or have dementia or physical impairment may be nonexistent, as medical providers may believe that the OAB problem is part of aging and solutions are not available. In certain cases treatment options can be limited for those impaired, and a caregiver, family member, or professional is the person most often responsible for carrying out the treatment plan or management strategies.

To make any impact on OAB and its management in older adults, it's important that caregivers have a clear view about the condition so that their care can be effective. Caregivers should:

- Understand physical and emotional harm that may result from a bladder control problem

- Demonstrate an understanding of OAB symptoms

- Consistently reinforce positive behavior

- Understand that success with rehabilitative behavioral treatments can occur

Home-Care Services

More and more, people are living into their eighties, nineties, and even hundreds! Many still live in their own homes, do their own cooking, and, for better or worse, drive their own cars. It's only human to want to stay in familiar surroundings, remain involved in community activities, and participate in family gatherings until the end of our days. Unfortunately, it's not always possible to maintain that independence. Unforeseen illness or disability and natural aging processes force many to seek physical care. When this situation arises, no one wants to go to a nursing home. That's why home care is the fastest-growing segment of the health care industry. The number of families providing long-term care to disabled and older parents and relatives is expected to increase substantially in the next few decades. Financially, home care is a better option than nursing-home care, as it can be provided at lower cost because the burden of caregiving lies with immediate and extended family members. As you become less independent, it is most likely that you'll be taken care of by a family member—your wife, daughter, daughter-in-law, or niece, as 75 percent of chronic home care is handled by women. Partners and spouses are the most common caregivers. Adult children and other family members usually only assume care responsibilities when a partner is absent.

As a concerned spouse or relative, how can you tell if your partner or family member is hiding an OAB problem? There are a few questions that may guide you:

- Is your family member unwilling to be away from home for more than one or two hours?

- Is there a sudden change in your family member's activity level?

- Do you smell urine in your family member's house or on their clothes?

- When your family member arrives at your house or at their destination, do they rush to the bathroom?

- Does your family member resist taking off a coat, suit jacket, or long sweater in public?

- Does your family member resist sitting down in social settings or sit "funny" in a chair?

- Does your family member purchase feminine hygiene pads, even after menopause?

If the answer to any of these questions is yes, you should talk with other family members about your suspicions of an OAB problem. Then seek assistance from a medical provider.

A couple may maintain a taboo against discussing OAB, despite their mutual awareness of the problem. A partner may be repelled by the stench on clothing and upholstery, yet say nothing in order to avoid humiliating the partner with OAB. A partner who refuses to perpetuate the silence and instead confides in family members may feel guilty for violating the other person's trust. However, once an OAB partner becomes ill, necessitating home caregiving, OAB becomes unbearable to both partners.

OAB can be a relentless source of weariness for caregivers, especially elderly caregivers. Physical exertion, often called "caregiver burden," increases day by day. People sometimes need to be lifted and turned to prevent skin breakdown, to change incontinence products, and to wash away the urine. And OAB is not only a daytime problem. During the night, a caregiver's sleep is usually disturbed to assist with toileting and transfers to commodes. There are situations where the caregiver's burden is so great that they become ill and, in the case of an elderly frail partner, may even die before the OAB person being cared for does.

Denial of OAB by an older family member is a tricky dilemma for both family members and medical providers who may be assisting the family with caregiving. Older people lose a degree of smell sensitivity as they age. Some block out their awareness of their OAB, particularly an incontinence problem, to avoid its implications. If the family confronts the denial head-on, they may provoke hostility and humiliation, causing people with OAB to further withdraw from acknowledging their problem.

If you're caring for a family member at home who is basically immobile and must always remain in bed, that person does not necessarily have to develop the OAB symptoms of incontinence. If getting out of bed to use the bathroom or bedside commode is not feasible, then offer a bedpan or urinal. Toileting is a private and personal act, so you need to be aware of the need for some privacy.

The following tips may help assist you toileting a family member:

♦ Try to give the person their own private bathroom so it's never being used by someone else. If a bathroom is inaccessible, use a bedside commode or urinal.

♦ Bed height should be sufficient so that when the person sits on the edge of the bed, their feet are flat and the person can easily accomplish moving from sitting to standing.

♦ Keep a clear, direct walking path to the toilet.

♦ Place night-lights along the path to bathroom.

♦ Make sure your family member can easily use the bathroom through the use of a raised toilet seat, grab bars, etc.

- ♦ Your family member should wear clothing that is easy to remove.

- ♦ Make sure the person empties their bladder before going to bed.

- ♦ Locate the bathroom when traveling, or carry a portable urinal. Choose seats in restaurants, theaters, etc. that are near a bathroom and on an aisle.

- ♦ Use underpads (reusable or disposable) under bedsheets, on chairs, and in the car. Avoid use of garbage bags, rubber pads, or shower liners, as these may be too slippery or may irritate skin.

- ♦ Open windows or use deodorizers to cut down on odors. A cut-up onion in a room will absorb odors without leaving its own smell. Also, an open box of baking soda will reduce odors.

Nocturia and nighttime incontinence can be a particular problem. Efforts should be made to maximize the sleep period. Sleep patterns change with age and become fragmented. There is a decreased amount of deep sleep and a higher percentage of more shallow sleep. Therefore, sleep occurs for shorter periods with many awakenings. To help the person minimize night urinating, follow the measures described in chapter 8.

OAB In The Nursing Home

The family of a person with OAB may eventually decide that home caregiving is too burdensome, and the person can no longer live at home. They may search for an alternative living arrangement that usually involves some form of community or group living. In many cases, caregivers will choose a nursing home in which to place their family member. The OAB symptom of urinary incontinence is a primary reason that precipitates or contributes to a person's decision to enter a nursing home or a family's decision to place an elder family member into nursing-home care. OAB is a common and expensive problem in nursing home residents, and there are many reasons for the problem. A decreased ability to move is an important factor, as nursing-home residents who are placed in restraints or in wheelchairs are unable to toilet when needed. Social indifference or mental incompetence also plays a role in the incidence of incontinence in nursing homes.

When Patrice visits her grandmother in Grove Nursing Home, she often finds her sitting in urine or stool. This really bothers Patrice, especially because Granny was always a meticulously clean person when she lived at home. At home, Granny was able to make it to the portable commode, which was kept close to her bed or chair. Granny knows when she has to urinate, but it comes on so quickly that she can't make it to the toilet in time. Patrice has discussed this with her grandmother, who says she doesn't want to be a bother to the staff because they are so busy with other residents who really need help. Granny says it's hard to go to the toilet on someone else's schedule.

As you can see from Patrice's experience, caregiving doesn't end when your family member enters a nursing home. It's just another phase of caregiving. It's still emotionally draining and still requires family involvement. Many people enter a nursing home able to maintain normal bladder function but lose their ability to use the toilet soon afterward, usually because they are in a strange environment and the staff fails to take them to the bathroom. Staff attitudes towards bladder control and incontinence play a major role in the way OAB residents are treated. Staff may act out negative feelings toward these residents by neglecting their needs.

Many nursing-home staff feel that residents are seeking secondary gains by being incontinent. The OAB resident correctly perceives that the only way to get attention, although many times negative attention, is through asking for assistance to the bathroom or being incontinent. Staff often believe that OAB is expected in nursing home residents because incontinence is a natural part of aging. They also often feel that it's quicker and easier to change an incontinence pad than it is to toilet a resident. This hopeless acceptance of OAB can make it into a "nonproblem." However, good care in nursing homes means that residents are toileted by staff according to an individualized care plan that has a specific schedule. Staff should also toilet residents upon request.

If the resident's OAB is a result of functional barriers, attention should be focused on urinating patterns so that toileting programs can be designed. If the resident can be rehabilitated, success may also be achieved with pelvic-muscle rehabilitation and bladder retraining. Patrice's grandmother is a perfect case for retraining. She knows when she has to urinate, but she can't hold it till the nurses can toilet her. She can be taught how to control the urge and to do some quick squeezes with her pelvic muscle. That may give her the control and time to wait for a nurse to help her. However, the staff needs to respond promptly to her requests for toileting. If retraining is not successful, then staff should start a scheduled toileting program. Consider David's story.

> *David has lived at the Trees Nursing Home for two years, ever since his wife died. David doesn't have any children or any relatives to speak of, and his only visitor is the pastor from his church. At times, David appears to be depressed. He recently was in the hospital for a heart problem. Since his return to the home, David lies in bed most of the day, especially after meals. Most times David is incontinent because he doesn't get himself out of bed fast enough to make it to the bathroom. The staff had a care-plan meeting and decided to place David on the following toileting schedule:*
>
> *6:30 A.M. Upon Awakening*
>
> *9:00 A.M. After Breakfast—encourage Allen to have a bowel movement*
>
> *11:00 A.M. Before Lunch*
>
> *1:30 P.M. Before Therapy*
>
> *3:30 P.M. After Therapy*
>
> *5:30 P.M. After Dinner*
>
> *8:00 P.M. Before Going to Bed*
>
> *11:00 P.M. Night Shift Staff*
>
> *In two weeks, David had decreased his urinary incontinent episodes to four or five times per week. The most significant change was that David asked to be toileted on a more consistent basis.*

Success stories like David's are achievable with a caring staff and nursing home administrative support.

Chances are you'll be caring for someone with OAB in the future. The caregiving does not need to be a burden. There are ways to manage the problem, allowing the person to remain independent and maintain a good quality of life.

Conclusion

Overactive bladder (OAB) is characterized by symptoms of urgency, usually with frequency and nocturia, with and without urge urinary incontinence. This bothersome medical condition affects men and women of all ages but is seen primarily in women. The incidence of OAB increases significantly with age and is a problem for millions of Americans. Most suffer in silence the embarrassment, inconvenience, and serious medical consequences of uncontrollable urges to urinate and the need to frequently access the bathroom. Their entire day centers around finding available toilets.

Every day, we, as medical providers, encounter women and men who are devastated by OAB. Most do not understand their OAB and its causes, don't know where to find answers, and are of the belief that there are no solutions. You may be one of these people—hiding your condition from your family, friends, and even from your doctor and other medical providers. If you suffer from OAB, it's important that you have all the facts.

Our aim for this book was to educate you about this bothersome bladder condition so you can become knowledgeable *before* seeking help. We want you to know that there is a very good possibility that you can overcome your problem. *Overcoming Overactive Bladder* presents the most current and accurate information on OAB. As you have probably realized, the treatments discussed require a commitment from you in order to be successful. These treatments require time and effort to be effective. We want you to think carefully about the options and find a medical provider who is knowledgeable about OAB so you can make good choices about your care. As a doctor and nurse, we believe the better informed person makes the best patient.

Appendix A

Manufacturers of Drugs and Products

This is a list of the major manufacturers of products, catheters, and devices for UI management. These manufacturers have additional educational material on OAB and their products.

3M Health Care
3M Center Bldg.
St. Paul, MN 55144-1000
(800) 228-3957
www.mmm.com/healthcare
Skin care and perineal cleanser products (brand name Cavilon, a no-sting barrier film)

Americare Products
115 Woodbine Lane
Danville, PA 17821
(800) 220-2273
www.aldanonline.com
Reusable pads and products

Aventis Pharmaceuticals
399 Interpace Parkway
Parsippany, NJ 07054
(800) 207-8049
www.avetispharma-us.com
DDAVP (demopressin)

Calmoseptine, Inc.
16602 Burke Lane
Huntington Beach, CA 92647
(800) 800-3405
www.calmoseptine.com
Skin-care ointment

Care-Tech Laboratories, Inc.
3224 South Kingshighway Blvd.
St. Louis, MO 63139
(800) 325-9681
www.caretechlabs.com
Skin care and perineal cleanser products (brand name Barri-Care)

Carrington Laboratories, Inc.
2001 Walnut Hill Lane
Irving, TX 75038
(800) 527-5216
www.carringtonlabs.com
Skin care, perineal cleanser, and deodorizer products (brand name Carrington)

Chester Labs, Inc.
1900 Section Road, Suite A
Cincinnati, OH 45237
(800) 354-9709
www.chester-labs.com
Skin Care products, perineal
cleansers, and odor eliminators
(brand name April Fresh)

Coloplast Corporation
1955 West Oak Circle
Marietta, GA 30062-2249
(800) 533-0464
www.us.coloplast.com
External catheters and drainage
bags (brand name Conveen),
skin care and perineal cleanser
products (brand name Baza)

Convatec
P.O. Box 5254
Princeton, NJ 08543-5254
(800) 422-8811
www.convatec.com
Skin care and perineal cleanser
products (brand names Aloe
Vesta and Sensi-Care)

DesChutes Medical Products, Inc.
1011 SW Emkay Drive, Suite 104
Bend, OR 97702
(800) 323-1363
www.deschutesmed.com
Pelvic muscle strengthening
devices (brand name Myself)

Dumex Medical
825 Franklin Court, Unit G
Marietta, GA 30067
(877) 796-8637
www.woundcaredirect.com
Skin care, perineal cleanser and
deodorizer products (brand
name PrimaDerm), reusable
absorbent pads and products.

E.K. Johnson
4869 G Street
Springfield, OR 97478
(541) 746-6126
Spill-proof rehab urinals

Eli Lilly and Company
Lilly Corporate Center
Indianapolis, Indiana 46285
(800) 545-5979
www.lilly.com
Duloxetine medication for SUI

Empi, Inc.
599 Cardigan Road
St. Paul, MN 55126-4099
(800) 450-3593
www.empi.com
Portable pelvic-floor muscle
exerciser and electrical
stimulation

First Quality Products, Inc.
80 Cuttermill Road, Suite 500
Great Neck, NY 11021
(800) 227-3551
www.fqnet.com
Disposable absorbent products.

Geri-Care Products
252 Wagner Street
Middlesex, NJ 08846
(732) 469-7722
www.geri-careproducts.com
Reusable absorbent products.

GOJO Industries. Inc,
One GOJO Plaza, Suite 500
Akron, OH 44311
(800) 321-9647
www.GOJO.com
Skin care and perineal cleanser
products (brand name Provon)

Healthpoint
2600 Airport Freeway
Fort Worth, TX 76111
(800) 441-8227
www.healthpoint.com
Skin care and perineal cleanser
and deodorizer products (brand
name Proshield)

Hollister, Inc.
InCare Medical Products
2000 Hollister Drive
Libertyville, IL 60048
(800) 323-4060
www.hollister.com
External male catheters and
pouches (for retracted penis),
external female pouches, catheter drainage bags, odor
eliminator products, skin care
(brand name Restore) and perineal cleansers. EMG/biofeed-
back equipment.

Humanicare International, Inc.
9 Elkins Road
North Brunswick, NJ 08816
(800) 631-5270
www.humanicare.com
Disposable and reusable absorbent products (brand name
Dignity)

Hygienics Industries
3968 194th Trail
Miami, FL 33160
(888) 463-7337
www.hygienics.com
Reusable absorbent products
(brand name Safe & Dry)

Indevus Pharmaceuticals, Inc.
99 Hayden Avenue, Suite 200
Lexington, MA 02421-7966
(800) 370-4742
www.indevus.com
Trospium chloride medication
for UUI and OAB

Kendall Confab Retail Group
601 Allendale Road
King of Prussia, PA 19406
(800) 326-6322
www.confab.com
Absorbent incontinence
products

Kimberly Clark Corporation
Adult Care Division
2001 Marathon Avenue
Neenah, WI 54956-9002
(888) 233-7363
www.depend.com or
www.poise.com
Retail supplier of absorbent
incontinence products (brand
name Depend)

Maddak, Inc.
6 Industrial Road
Pequannock, NJ 07440
(973) 628-7600
www.maddak.com
Bathroom toileting aids

Mallinckrodt Inc.
675 McDonnell Blvd.
St Louis, MO 63134
(888) 744-1414
www.mallinckrodt.com
Tofranil (imipramine HCL)

McKesson Medical-Surgical
8741 Landmark Road
Richmond, VA 23228
(800) 446-3008
www.mckgenmed.com
Skin cleansers, creams (brand name StayDry) and absorbent products

Medtronic
800 53rd Avenue, NE
Minneapolis, MN 55421
(800) 328-0810
www.interstim.com
Implantable electrical stimulator (brand name Interstim)

Mentor Healthcare-Urology
201 Mentor Drive
Santa Barbara, CA 93111
(800) 328-3863
www.mentorcorp.com
External catheters and pessaries

Milex Products, Inc.
4311 North Normandy Avenue
Chicago, IL 60634-1403
(800) 621-1278
www.milexproducts.com
Pessaries and vaginal weights

Novartis Pharmaceuticals
608 Fifth Avenue
New York, NY 10020
(212) 307-1122
www.novartis.org
Darifenacin (trade name Enablex) for OAB

Ortho-McNeil Pharmaceutical
1000 Rt. 202, Box 300
Raritan, NJ 08869
(888) 395-1232
www.ditropanxl.com
Oxybutynin chloride (brand name Ditropan XL)

Paper-Pak Products, Inc.
1941 White Avenue
LaVerne, CA 91750
(800) 635-4560
www.paperpak.com
Disposable absorbent products (brand name Confidence)

Pfizer Corporation
235 East 42nd Street
New York, NY 10017
(866) 420-9400
www.detrolla.com
Tolterodine tartrate (brand name Detrol), estrogen vaginal tablets (brand name Vagifem), vaginal ring (brand name Estring)

Principle Business Enterprises
P.O. Box 129
Dunbridge, OH 43414-0129
(800) 467-3224
www.gopeach.com
Disposable absorbent products (brand name Tranquility)

Salk Company, Inc.
119 Braintree Street
P.O. Box 452
Boston, MA 02134
(888) 289-7255
www.salkcompany.com
Disposable absorbent products (brand name Salk Select)

SCA Incontinence Care
500 Baldwin Tower
Eddystone, PA 19022
(800) 992-9939
www.tena-usa.com
Disposable absorbent products (brand name Tena), skin cleansers

Smith & Nephew, Inc.
11775 Starkey Road
Largo, FL 33773-1970
(800) 876-1261
www.snwmd.com
Skin care products (brand name
Triple Care), cleansers

Standard Textile Company
1 Knollcrest Drive
P.O. Box 371805
Cincinnati, OH 45222-1805
(800) 999-0400
www.standardtextile.com
Reusable absorbent products

Sunrise Medical, Inc.
7477 East Dry Creek Parkway
Longmont, CO 80503
(800) 333-4000
www.standardtextile.com
Raised toilet seats

Swiss-American Products, Inc.
4641 Nall Road
Dallas, TX 75244
(800) 633-8872
www.elta.net
Skin care products (brand name
Elta)

Utah Medical Products, Inc.
7043 South 300 West
Midvale, UT 84047
(800) 533-4984
www.utahmed.com
Pelvic-floor electrical stimulator

Warner Chilcott Company
Consumer Healthcare
201 Tabor Road
Morris Plains, NJ 07950
(800) 524-2624
www.estrace.com
vaginal cream (brand name
Estrace)

Watson Pharma, Inc.
360 Mt. Kemble Avenue
P.O. Box 1953
Morristown, NJ 07962-1953
(888) 699-7765
www.oxytrol.com
transdermal patch (brand name
Oxytrol)

Wyeth-Ayerst Laboratories
Division of Home Products Corp
P.O. Box 8299
Philadelphia, PA 19101
(800) 999-9284
www.premarin.com
oral, patch, vaginal cream
(brand name Premarin)

Yamanouchi Pharma America, Inc.
61 South Paramus Road, 4th Floor
Paramus, NJ 07652
(201) 291-2556
www.yamanouchiamerica.com
Solifenacin (brand name
Vesicare)

Mail-Order Catalogs

These companies will send you catalogs upon request

Byram Healthcare Centers, Inc.
Home Health Supplies
11400 47th Street North, Suite A
Clearwater, FL 33762
(800) 354-4054 (CT, NY, NJ)
(800) 649-9882 (MA, VT, RI, ME)
(800) 234-1779 (All other states)

Edgepark Surgical Inc.
1810 Summit Commerce Park
Twinsburg, OH 44087
(800) 321-0591
www.edgepark.com

Home Delivery Incontinent
Supplies Co., Inc. (HDIS)
9385 Dielman Industrial Drive
Olivette, MO 63132
(800) 269-4663
www.hdis.com

Appendix B

Self-Help Groups and Resources

The following groups can be contacted for more information on OAB.

Agency for Healthcare Research and Quality (formerly Agency for Health Care Policy and Research)
P.O. Box 8547
Silver Spring, MD 20852
(301) 594-1364
www.ahrq.gov

Alliance for Aging
2021 K Street, NW, Suite 305
Washington, DC 20006
(202) 293-2856
www.agingresearch.org

American College of Obstetricians and Gynecology (ACOG)
409 12th, SW
Washington, DC 20024
(202) 638-5577
www.acog.com

American Foundation of Urologic Disease (AFUD)
300 W. Pratt, Suite 401
Baltimore, MD 21201-2463
(800) 242-2383
www.afud.com

American Physical Therapy Association
Section on Women's Health
111 N. Fairfax Street
Alexandria, VA 22314
(703) 684-2782
www.APTA.org

Association of Women's Health, Obstetric and Neonatal Nurses
2000 L Street, NW, Suite 740
Washington DC 20036
(800) 673-8499
www.awhonn.org

American Urogynecologic Society (AUGS)
2025 M Street NW, Suite 800
Washington DC 20036
(202) 367-1167
www.augs.org

American Urological Association (AUA)
1120 N. Charles Street
Baltimore, MD 21201
(410) 727-1100
www.auanet.org

International Foundation for Functional Gastrointestinal Disorders
P.O. Box 170864
Milwaukee, WI 53217-8076
(414) 964-1799
www.iffgd.com

National Association For Continence (NAFC)
P.O. Box 1019
385 Meeting Street, Suite 100
Charleston, SC 29402
(800) BLADDER (800-252-3337)
www.nafc.org

National Institute of Diabetes and Digestive and Kidney Diseases (NIDDK)
National Institutes of Health
Westwood Building, Suite 3A-05
Bethesda, MD 20892
www.niddk.nih.gov

Simon Foundation for Continence
Box 835-F
Wilmette, IL 60092
(800) 237-4666
www.simonfoundation.com

Society of Urologic Nurses and Associates (SUNA)
East Holy Avenue, Box 56
Pitman, NJ 09071-0056
(888) TAP-SUNA (888-827-7862)
www.suna.org

US-TOO International, Inc.
Prostate Cancer Survivor
Support Groups
5003 Fairview Avenue
Downers Grove, IL 60515
(800) 808-7866
www.ustoo.org

Wellness Partners, LLC
237 Old Tilton Road
Canterbury, NH 03224
www.seekwellness.com

Wound, Ostomy and Continence Nurses Society (WOCN)
4700 West Lake Avenue
Glenview, IL 60025
(800) 224-9626
www.wocn.org

Glossary of Commonly Used Terms

Absorbent incontinence products: Pads and garments, either disposable or reusable, worn to contain urinary incontinence or uncontrolled urine leakage. Absorbent products include shields, guards, undergarment pads, combination pad-pant systems, diaper-like garments, and bed pads.

Acetylcholine: One of the chemicals (referred to as a neurotransmitter) that plays an important part in the transmission of nerve impulses in the parasympathetic nervous system. This chemical cause the bladder muscle (detrusor) to squeeze or contract.

Abdomen (referred to as "belly"): Area of the body between the lower border of the ribs and upper border of the thighs.

Anal sphincters: Two rings of the pelvic-floor muscle that surround the rectum and anus, which help control passage of bowel movements.

Antibiotics: Substances that inhibit the growth of or kill microorganisms (bacteria) and that are used to treat infections.

Anticholinergics: A drug that interferes with the effects of acetylcholine thus decreasing the action of the parasympathetic nervous system. An anticholinergic drug will aid the bladder in storage of urine by increasing bladder capacity and decreasing bladder overactivity.

Anus: The final two inches of the rectum, surrounded by the internal anal sphincter and the external sphincter.

Bacteria: Microscopic organisms that can cause infection and are usually treated with antibiotics.

Bacteriuria: Bacteria present in the urine in a minimum of 100,000 colony forming units (cfu) per mL.

Bedside commode: A portable toilet used by individuals who have difficulty getting to standard facilities.

Behavioral treatments: Specific interventions designed to alter the relationship between the person's symptoms and their behavior and/or environment for the treatment of OAB.

Benign prostatic hyperplasia (BPH): A common disorder of men over the age of fifty, characterized by enlargement of the prostate which may press against the urethra and interfere with the flow of urine causing overflow incontinence. BPH is the most common cause of such anatomic obstruction in elderly men.

Biofeedback therapy: A behavioral technique in which a person learns how to consciously control responses such as muscle contractions. The person receives a visual, auditory, or tactile signal (the feedback) that indicates how well the person's muscles are responding to the commands of the person's nervous system.

Bladder: A balloon-like organ located in the pelvis. The bladder has only two functions: to stretch to allow the storage of urine and to contract to enable the expulsion of urine. The term "detrusor" is used to refer to the smooth muscle structure of the bladder.

Bladder diary or record: A daily record of bladder habits that includes the frequency, timing, urgency, and/or other factors associated with a person's urinating.

Bladder training: A behavioral technique that requires the patient to resist or inhibit the sensation of urgency (the strong desire to urinate), to postpone urinating, and to urinate according to a timetable rather than to the urge to urinate.

Bowel movement: The act of passing feces through the anus.

Bowels: Another word for intestines.

Cholinergic: Fibers in the parasympathetic nervous system that release acetylcholine.

Condom catheters: A condom like device placed over the penis to allow bladder drainage and collection of urine.

Constipation: Infrequent or difficult passing of hard and dry feces or stool.

Continence: The ability to voluntarily control urination or defecation until an appropriate time and place can be found.

Cystitis: Irritation or inflammation (swelling) of the bladder usually caused by an infection.

Cystocele: An intrusion or bulging of the bladder into the vagina, usually caused when the vaginal muscles that support the bladder and urethra are stretched or damaged.

Daytime frequency: The number of times urination is recorded during waking hours and includes the first urination after waking and rising in the morning.

Defecation: The act of emptying the bowels or having a bowel movement.

Detrusor: The large muscle in the bladder that stretches to store urine and squeezes or contracts to expel the urine. This muscle may be too active in people with OAB.

Diuretic: An agent (like drugs, alcohol, or caffeine) that increases urination by causing the kidneys to secrete more fluid from the blood.

Dribbling: refers to urine loss after completion of urination.

Enuresis: The involuntary loss of urine (urinary incontinence).

Estrogen: A hormone produced primarily by the ovaries. Estrogen is believed to play a major role in maintaining the strength and tone of the pelvic floor.

Evacuation: Another word for bowel movement.

External sphincter: Band of muscle downstream from the internal sphincter responsible for maintaining urinary and fecal continence.

Fecal incontinence: The accidental and involuntary loss of liquid, solid stool, or gas from the anus.

Feces: Waste material from the intestines. Feces, also referred to as "stool," are composed of bacteria, undigested food, and material sloughed from the intestines.

Frequency: Urinating more than eight times in a twenty-four-hour period, including two or more times at night.

Hematuria: Blood in the urine, which may only be detected under the microscope.

Hesitancy: A difficulty or delay in initiating urination resulting in delay in the onset of urination after the person is ready to pass urine.

Incontinence: The accidental or unwanted loss of urine or feces. A person may have urinary or fecal incontinence or both (sometimes called double incontinence).

Kegel exercises: Exercises to strength the pelvic-floor and sphincter muscles, named after Dr. Arnold Kegel, who first prescribed a specific set of pelvic floor exercises to women in the 1940s.

Kidneys: A pair of bean-shaped urine-making organs that are located behind the eleventh and twelfth ribs. Their principal function is to filter the blood to separate out waste products, which are combined with excess water to form urine.

Levator ani: Anterior portion of the pubococcygeus muscle.

Lower urinary tract: Consists of the bladder, prostate gland (in men), urethra, and urinary sphincters.

LUTS: Abbreviation for "lower urinary-tract symptoms," which is a group of symptoms which include, incontinence, weak stream, hesitancy, urgency of urination, frequency, nocturia, posturination dribbling, and intermittency, or an interrupted urinary stream.

Meatus: The opening to the urethra.

Micturition: Another term for urination.

Nervous system: The voluntary and involuntary nervous systems are composed of the brain, the spinal cord, and the sensory nerves that provide messages to the brain from the body, and motor nerves, which provide messages from the brain to the muscles organs.

Nighttime frequency: Complaint of needing to urinate one or more times per night between the time the person goes to bed with the intention of sleeping and the time the person wakes with the intention of rising.

Nocturia: Waking up two or more times at night because of the need or urge to urinate.

Nocturnal enuresis: Complaint of loss of urine during sleep. In children it is called bedwetting.

Parasympathetic nerves: "Maintenance" component of the autonomic nervous system. Stimulation of the parasympathetic nervous system innervating the bladder promotes voiding by stimulating the bladder muscle to contract, causing the urge sensation and indirectly relaxing the internal urethral sphincter, which allows urine to enter the urethra. Stimulation of the parasympathetic nervous system pathways innervating the intestinal tract increase motility and secretion.

Pelvic muscles (often referred to as pelvic floor): General term referring to the muscles of the pelvic diaphragm and urogenital diaphragm as one unit. These muscles form a "hammock," slung from the front of the pelvis to the end of the spinal cord or cocyx. They support the organs of the pelvis, the bladder, uterus, and the rectum.

Pelvic-muscle exercises (PMEs): A behavioral treatment that requires repetitive active exercise of the pubococcygeus muscle to improve urethral resistance and urinary control by strengthening the periurethral and pelvic muscles. Also called Kegel exercises, pelvic-floor exercises, or pelvic-floor muscle training.

Pelvis: The ring of bones at the lower end of the trunk in which the pelvic organs are housed.

Perineum: Area between the anus and vagina in women, and anus and base of penis in men.

Pessary: Devices for women that are placed in the vagina to treat pelvic relaxation or prolapse of pelvic organs.

Prolapse: To slide forward or downward usually referring to the pelvic organs, such as the falling down of the bladder, uterus, or rectum through the vagina.

Prostate: A walnut-shaped gland found in men that surrounds the urethra between the bladder and the pelvic floor.

Prostatitis: Irritation or inflammation of the prostate.

Prostatectomy: Surgical removal of part or all of the prostate.

Pubococcygeus muscle: Another name for the levator ani muscle, one of the pelvic muscles that hold the pelvic organs in place.

Pudendal nerve: Main nerve supplying the pelvic floor, bladder and urethra. Damage to this nerve can cause incontinence.

Rectocele: Bulging of the rectum into the space normally occupied by the vagina, suggesting weakness of the pelvic floor.

Rectum: Last segment of colon, or large intestine; the lowest part of the bowel, found right before the anus.

Retention: Inability to empty urine from the bladder, which can be caused by atonic bladder or obstruction of the urethra.

Sphincter: A ring of muscle around a natural opening or passage that acts like a valve controlling in this case the flow of urine out of the body.

Sacral nerve stimulation: A surgical procedure that implants a pacemaker device at the base of the spinal cord and is used to treat severe OAB symptoms of urgency and frequency.

Stress urinary incontinence: The involuntary loss of urine from the urethra during effort or physical exertion; for example, during coughing and laughing.

Suprapubic: Above the pubic bone.

Sympathetic nerves: "Fight or flight" components of the autonomic nervous system, which originate in the thoracic and lumbar region of the spinal cord. Stimulation of the sympathetic innervating the bladder promotes bladder filling by relaxing the bladder (detrusor) muscle and contracting the internal proximal portion of the urethral sphincter to prevent urine from entering the urethra. Sympathetic fibers innervating the intestine cause reduced motility and reduced secretions.

Topical: When a medication (like a cream or ointment) is applied to a specific site or location, usually on the skin or external part of the body.

Trigone: Triangle-shaped part of the bladder that extends up from the urethra, up to the posterior bladder wall, to the ureteral openings.

Ureters: Two very thin muscular tubes, about eight or nine inches long, through which urine flows from the kidneys to the bladder.

Urethra: A narrow tube that carries urine from the bladder outside of the body during urination. The opening of the urethra is at the end of the penis in men and just above the vaginal opening in women.

Urethrocele: A prolapse or falling down of the urethra into the vaginal wall.

Urge: The sensation from the bladder producing the desire to urinate.

Urge urinary incontinence: The involuntary and accidental loss of urine when a person is aware of the need to get to the bathroom but is not able to hold the urine long enough to get there. Usually it is immediately preceded by urgency.

Urgency: A strong, intense, and often sudden desire to urinate.

Urinary incontinence (UI): Unwanted or accidental loss (leakage) of urine.

Urinary system: Part of the body (kidneys, ureters, bladder, and urethra) that produces, stores, and eliminates urine.

Urinary tract: Body system that makes, stores, and releases urine, it includes the ureters, bladder, and urethra.

Urinate: To void or to pass urine.

Urination: The act of passing urine.

Urine: A mixture of waste products and water produced by the kidneys.

Uterine prolapse: When the uterus has slipped (dropped) from its normal position and the cervix is lower in or may protrude outside the vagina.

Vagina: Also known as the birth canal. The vagina is a collapsible tube of smooth muscle with its opening located between the urethral orifice and the anal sphincter of women.

Void: See Urinate.

References

Abrams, P., R. Freeman, C. Anderstrom, and A. Mattiasson. 1998. Tolterodine, a new antimuscarinic agent: as effective but better tolerated than oxybutynin in patients with an overactive bladder. *British Journal of Urology* 81:801–810.

Abrams P., L. Cardozo, M. Fall, D. Griffiths, P. Rosier, U. Ulmsten, et.al. 2002. The standardization of terminology of lower urinary tract function. *Neurourology and Urodynamics* 21:167-178.

Anderson, R., D. Mobley, B. Blank, D. Saltzman, J. Susset, and J. Brown. 1999. Once daily controlled versus immediate-release oxybutynin chloride for urge urinary incontinence. *The Journal of Urology* 161:1809–1812.

Appell, R., M. Chancellor, H. Zobrist, H. Thomas, and S. Sanders. 2003. Pharmacokinetics, metabolism and saliva output during transdermal and extended-release oral oxybutynin administration in healthy subjects. *Mayo Clinical Proceedings* 78:696-702.

Arya L., D. Myers, and N.D. Jackson. 2000. Dietary caffeine intake and the risk for detrusor instability: a case-control study. *Obstetrics & Gynecology* 96(1):85-89

Bass, D., M. Prevo, and D. Waxman. 2002. Gastrointestinal safety of an extended-release, nondeformable oral dosage form (OROSÒ), a retrospective study. *Drug Safety* 25(14):1021-1033.

Brown, J., E. Vittinghoff, J. Wyman, K. Stone, M. Nevitt, K. Ensrud, et al. 2000. Urinary incontinence: does it increase risk for falls and fracture? *Journal of American Geriatrics Society* 48:721-725.

Brown, J. 2002. Epidemiology and changing demographics of overactive bladder: A focus on the postmenopausal women. *Urology Times* 30(Suppl 2):6-11.

Brown, J., W. McGhan, and S. Chokroverty. 2001. Comorbidities associated with overactive bladder. *American Journal of Managed Care* 9(Suppl):S574-S579.

Burgio, K., P. Goode, J. Locher, M. Umlauf, D. Roth, H. Richter, et.al. 2002. Behavioral training with and without biofeedback in the treatment of urge incontinence in older women. *Journal of the American Medical Association* 288(18):2293-2299.

Burgio, K., J. Locher, P. Goode, M. Hardin, B. McDowell, M. Dombrowski, and D. Candib. 1998. Behavioral vs. drug treatment for urge urinary incontinence in older women. *Journal of the American Medical Association* (23):1995-1999

Burgio, K., J. Locher, and P. Goode. 2000 Combined behavioral and drug therapy for urge incontinence in older women. *Journal of American Geriatric Society* 48:370-374.

Burgio, K., K. Lynette, Pearce, and A. Lucco. 1989. *Staying Dry, A Practical Guide to Bladder Control*, Baltimore: The Johns Hopkins University Press.

Burnett, A., W. G. Davila, D. Newman, and S. Hardestry. 2002. Clinical and Cost-Effective Strategies in the Management of Urinary Incontinence. *Managed Care Consultant* 5-39.

Cannon, T. W., and M. B. Cancellor. 2002. Pharmacotherapy of the overactive bladder and advances in drug delivery. *Clin Obstet Gynecol* 45(1):205-217

Chancellor M., S. Freedman, H. Mitcheson, J. Antoci, G. Primus, and A. Wein. 2000. Tolterodine, an effective and well-tolerated treatment for urge incontinence and other overactive bladder symptoms. *Clinical Drug Investigations* 19:83–91.

Chapple C. R., T. Yamanishi, and R. Chess-Williams. 2002. Muscarinic receptor subtypes and management of the overactive bladder. *Urology.* 60(Suppl 5A):82-89.

Davila, W. G., C. Daugherty, and S. Sanders. 2001. A short-term, multicenter, randomized double-blind dose titration study of the efficacy and anticholinergic side effects of transdermal compared to immediate release oral oxybutynin treatment of patients with urge urinary incontinence. *The Journal of Urology* 166(1):140-145.

DuBeau, C. 2002. The continuum of urinary incontinence in an aging population. *Urology Times* 30(suppl 2):12-17.

Dierich, M, and F. Froe. 2000. *Overcoming Incontinence.* New York: John Wiley & Sons, Inc.

Diokno, A., R. Appell, P. Sand, R. Dmochowski, B. Gburek, I. Klimberg, and S. Kell. 2003. Prospective, randomized, double-blind study of the efficacy and tolerability of the extended-release formulations of oxybutynin and tolterodine for overactive bladder: results of the OPERA trial. *Mayo Clinical Proceedings* 78:687-695.

Dmochowski, R., W. G. Davila, N. Zinner, M. Gittelman, D. Saltzstein, S. Lyttle, and S. Sanders. 2002. Efficacy and safety of transdermal oxybutynin in patients with urge and mixed incontinence. *The Journal of Urology* 168(2):580-586.

Dmochowski R. R., J. R. Miklos, P. A. Norton, and N. R. Zinner. 2003. Duloxetine versus placebo for the treatment of North American women with stress urinary incontinence. *The Journal of Urology* 170:1259-1263.

Dugan, E., S. Cohen, D. Bland, J. Preisser, C. Davis, P. Suggs, and P. McGann. 2000. The association of depressive symptoms and urinary incontinence among older adults. *Journal of American Geriatric Society* 48:413-416.

Duong T., and A. Korn. 2001. A comparison of urinary incontinence among African-American, Asian, Hispanic and white women. *American Journal Obstetric Gynecology* 184(6):1083-6.

Fultz N., A. Herzog, R. Regula, R. Wallace, and A. Diokno. 1999. Prevalence and severity of urinary incontinence in older African American and Caucasian women. *Journal of Gerontology Medical Science* 54A(6):M299-M303.

Gupta, S. K., and G. Sathyan. 1999. Pharmacokinetics of an oral once-a-day controlled-release oxybutynin formulation compared with immediate-release oxybutynin. *J Clin Pharmacol* 39(3):289-296.

Hall, J., M. Nelson, J. Meyer, T. Williamson, and S. Wagner. 2001. Costs and resources associated with the treatment of overactive bladder using retrospective medical care claims data. *Managed Care Interface* 8:69-75.

Hampel, C., D. Wienhold, N. Benken, C. Egersmann, and J. Thuroff. 1997 Definition of overactive bladder and epidemiology of urinary incontinence. *Urology* 50:4-14.

Hu, T. W., and T. Wagner. 2001. Economic considerations in overactive bladder. *American Journal of Managed Care* 6:S591-598.

Hu T. W., T. H. Wagner, and J. D. Bentkover. 2003. Estimated economic costs of overactive bladder in the United States. *Urology.* 61:1123-1128.

Kelleher, C. 2002. Economic and social impact of OAB. *European Urology Supplements* 1:11-16.

Kobelt G., I. Kirchberger, and J. Malone-Lee. 1999. Quality of life aspects of the overactive bladder and the effect of treatment with tolterodine. *British Journal Urology International* 83:583-90.

Kuo, H. C. 2003. Effectiveness of intravesical resiniferatoxin for anticholinergic treatment refractory detrusor overactive due to nonspinal cord lesions. *The Journal of Urology* 170:835-839.

Lacey, J., P. Mink, J. Lubin, M. Sherman, R. Troisi, P. Hartge, A. Schatzkin, and C. Schairer. 2002. Menopausal hormone replacement therapy and risk of ovarian cancer. *Journal of the American Medical Association* 288:334-341.

Langa, K., N. Fultz, S. Saint, M. Kabeto, and R. Herzog. 2002. Informal caregiving time and costs for urinary incontinence in older individuals in the United States. *Journal of American Geriatrics Society* 50:733-737.

Lapitan, M., and P. Chye. 2001. The epidemiology of overactive bladder among females in Asia: a questionnaire survey. *International Urogynecology Journal* 12:226-231.

Liberman, J., et al. 2001. Health-related quality of life among adults with symptoms of overactive bladder: results from a U.S. community based survey. *Urology* 57:1044-1050.

Linder, M. 2003. *Void Where Prohibited*. Iowa City. Fanpihua Press.

Luber, K., S. Boero, and J. Choe. 2001. The demographics of pelvic floor disorders: current observations and future projections. *American Journal Obstetric Gynecology* 184:1496-1501.

Lustbader, W., and N. Hooyman. 1994. *Taking Care of Aging Family Member*. New York: The Free Press.

Madersbacher H., M. Stohrer, R. Richter, et al. 1995. Trospium chloride versus oxybutynin: a randomized, double-blind, multicenter trial in the treatment of detrusor hyper-reflexia. *British Journal Urology* 75:452-456.

Murphy M, A. J. Carmichael. 2000. Transdermal drug delivery systems and skin sensitivity reactions. Incidence and management. *Am J Clin Dermatol.* 1:361-368.

Milsom, I., P. Abrams, L. Cardozo, R. Roberts, J. Thuroff, and A. Wein. 2001. How widespread are the symptoms of an overactive bladder and how are they managed? A population-based prevalence study. *British Journal Urology International* 87:760-766.

Newman, D. 2003. Stress urinary incontinence in women. *American Journal Nursing* 103(8):46-55.

———. 2002. *Managing and Treating Urinary Incontinence*. Baltimore: Health Professions Press.

———. 1999 *The Urinary Incontinence Sourcebook* (2nd edition). Los Angeles: Lowell House.

Newman, D., and D. Giovanni. 2002. Overactive bladder: A nursing perspective. *American Journal of Nursing* 102(6):36-46.

Newman, D., and M. Palmer. 2003. State of the science on urinary incontinence. *American Journal of Nursing*, 3[Suppl]:1-53.

Nilvebrant L. 2000. The mechanism of action of tolterodine. *Review Contempory Pharmacotherapy* 11:13–27.

Norton, P., N. Zinner, I. Yalcin, and R. Bump. 2002. Duloxetine versus placebo in the treatment of stress urinary incontinence. *American Journal Obstetrics Gynecology* 187(1):40-48.

Nygaard I., and M. Linder. 1997. Thirst at work; an occupational hazard? *International Urogynecology Journal* 8(6):340-343.

Palmer, M., S. Fitzgerald, S. Berry, and K. Hart. 1999. Urinary incontinence in working women: an exploratory study. *Women and Health* 29(3):67-80.

Parker, W., A. Rosenman, and R. Parker. 2002. *The Incontinence Solution*. New York: Simon & Shuster, Inc.

Ricci, J., J. Baggish, T. Hunt, W. Stewart, A. Wein, R. A. Herzog, A. Diokno. 2001. Coping strategies and healthcare-seeking behavior in a U.S. national sample of adults with symptoms suggestive of overactive bladder. *Clinical Therapeutics* 23(8):1245-1259.

Roe, B., H. Doll, and K. Wilson. 1999. Help-seeking behaviour and health and social services utilization by people suffering from urinary incontinence. *International Journal of Nursing Studies* 36:245-253.

Rovner, E., A. Wein, and D. Caruso. 2002. *A Woman's Guide to Regaining Bladder Control*. New York: M. Evans and Co., Inc.

Shah D, and G. Badlani. 2002. Treatment of overactive bladder and incontinence in the elderly. *Rev Urol* 4(Suppl 4):S38-S43.

Stewart W., R. Herzog, and A. Wein. 2001. The prevalence and impact of overactive bladder in the U.S.: results from the NOBLE program. *Neurourology Urodynamics* 20:406-408.

Stewart, W. F., J. B. Van Roover, G. W. Cundiff, et al. 2003. Prevalence and burden of overactive bladder in the United States. *World J Urol* 20(6):237-336.

Thor K., and M. Katofiasc. 1995. Effects of duloxetine, a combined serotonin and norepinephrine reuptake inhibitor, on central neural control of lower urinary tract function in the choralose-anesthetized female cat. *Journal Pharmacology Exp Ther* 274(2): 1014-24.

Tomlinson, B., M. Dougherty, J. Pendergast, A. Boyington, M. Coffman, and S. Pickens. 1999. Dietary caffeine, fluid intake and urinary incontinence in older rural women. *International Urogynecology Journal* 10:22-28.

Van Kerrebroeck, P., K. Kreder, U. Jonas, N. Zinner, and A. Wein. 2001. On behalf of the Tolterodine Study Group. Tolterodine once-daily: Superior efficacy and tolerability in the treatment of the overactive bladder. *Urology* 57(3):414-421.

Versi, E., R. Appell, D. Mobley, W. Patton, and D. Saltzstein. 2000. Dry mouth with conventional and controlled-release oxybutynin in urinary incontinence. *Obstetrics & Gynecology* 95:718–721.

Viktrup, L., and G. Lose. 2001. The risk of stress incontinence 5 years after first delivery. *American Journal of Obstetrics & Gynecology* 185(1):82-87.

Voytas, J. 2002. The role of geriatricians and family practitioners in the treatment of overactive bladder and incontinence. *Reviews in Urology* 2(4):S44-S49.

Wein, A. 2001. Pharmacological agents for the treatment of urinary incontinence due to overactive bladder. *Expert Opinion on Investigational Drugs* 10(1):65-83.

Wein A., and E. Rovner. 2002. Definition and epidemiology of overactive bladder. *Urology* 60:7-12.

———. 2002. The treatment of overactive bladder in the geriatric patient. *Clinical Geriatrics* 10(1):1-12.

———. 1999. The overactive bladder: An overview for primary care health providers. *International Journal of Fertility* 44(2):56-66.

Wein A., and R. Roberts. 2000. Overactive bladder survey evaluates the extent of symptoms in family doctor setting. *Family Urology* 5:7-8.

Wyman, J., and A. J. Fantl. 1991. Bladder training in ambulatory care management of urinary incontinence. *Urologic Nursing* 11:11-17.

Yarker E., et al. 1999. Oxybutynin: a review of its pharmacodynamics and pharmacokinetic properties, and its therapeutic use in detrusor instability. *Drugs and Aging* 6:243–262.

Zorn, B., H. Montgomery, K. Pieper, M. Gray, and W. Steers. 1999. Urinary incontinence and depression. *Journal of Urology* 162:82-4.

Some Other
New Harbinger Titles

Eating Mindfully, Item 3503, $13.95

Living with RSDS, Item 3554 $16.95

The Ten Hidden Barriers to Weight Loss, Item 3244 $11.95

The Sjogren's Syndrome Survival Guide, Item 3562 $15.95

Stop Feeling Tired, Item 3139 $14.95

Responsible Drinking, Item 2949 $18.95

The Mitral Valve Prolapse/Dysautonomia Survival Guide, Item 3031 $14.95

Stop Worrying Abour Your Health, Item 285X $14.95

The Vulvodynia Survival Guide, Item 2914 $15.95

The Multifidus Back Pain Solution, Item 2787 $12.95

Move Your Body, Tone Your Mood, Item 2752 $17.95

The Chronic Illness Workbook, Item 2647 $16.95

Coping with Crohn's Disease, Item 2655 $15.95

The Woman's Book of Sleep, Item 2493 $14.95

The Trigger Point Therapy Workbook, Item 2507 $19.95

Fibromyalgia and Chronic Myofascial Pain Syndrome, second edition, Item 2388 $19.95

Kill the Craving, Item 237X $18.95

Rosacea, Item 2248 $13.95

Thinking Pregnant, Item 2302 $13.95

Shy Bladder Syndrome, Item 2272 $13.95

Help for Hairpullers, Item 2329 $13.95

Coping with Chronic Fatigue Syndrome, Item 0199 $13.95

Call **toll free, 1-800-748-6273,** or log on to our online bookstore at **www.newharbinger.com** to order. Have your Visa or Mastercard number ready. Or send a check for the titles you want to New Harbinger Publications, Inc., 5674 Shattuck Ave., Oakland, CA 94609. Include $4.50 for the first book and 75¢ for each additional book, to cover shipping and handling. (California residents please include appropriate sales tax.) Allow two to five weeks for delivery.

Prices subject to change without notice.